Cancer Etiology, Diagnosis and Treatments

The Revolution of Robotic Stereotactic Radiotherapy (Robotic Radiosurgery) in Lung Cancer

CANCER ETIOLOGY, DIAGNOSIS AND TREATMENTS

Additional books in this series can be found on Nova's website under the Series tab.

Additional e-books in this series can be found on Nova's website under the e-book tab.

CANCER ETIOLOGY, DIAGNOSIS AND TREATMENTS

THE REVOLUTION OF ROBOTIC STEREOTACTIC RADIOTHERAPY (ROBOTIC RADIOSURGERY) IN LUNG CANCER

PIERRE-YVES BONDIAU, M.D., Ph.D.
EDITOR

New York

For permission to use material from this book please contact us:
Telephone 631-231-7269; Fax 631-231-8175
Web Site: http://www.novapublishers.com

Library of Congress Cataloging-in-Publication Data

ISBN: 978-1-62808-718-5
Library of Congress Control Number: 2014942198

Published by Nova Science Publishers, Inc. † New York

Contents

Part I: Lung Cancer

In: The Revolution of Robotic …
Editor: Pierre-Yves Bondiau
ISBN: 978-1-62808-718-5

Chapter 1

Introduction to Stereotactic Body Radiotherapy

***Pierre-Yves Bondiau**1,2 *and Eric F. Lartigau*†3**
1 Department of Radiation Oncology,
Antoine-Lacassagne Cancer Center, Nice, France
2 University of Nice Sophia-Antipolis, Nice, France.
3 Department of Radiation Oncology,
Oscar Lambret Cancer Center and University Lille II, Lille, France

From 2D to 3D Radiotherapy

Since the start of the century, the gold standard for stage I (T1-2, N0) NSCLC is surgical resection giving a five years survival rate of 60% to70%. For medically inoperable patients, an alternative is radiotherapy. In the 70's, radiotherapy was done in 2Dimension, the field of irradiation including primary tumor and regional lymphatics in the ipsilateral hilum and mediastinum. These treatments were poorly tolerated and in a study reported by Sibley [1], 156 patients with Stage I medically inoperable with non-small–cell lung cancer, were treated by 2D Radiotherapy (2DRT). There were 54% T1N0 and 46% T2N0. Median dose delivered to the target was 64 Gy (50 to 80 Gy) with a median size of the target of 3 cm (range 0.5 to 8). Results for the

* Email: pierre-yves.bondiau@nice.unicancer.fr.
† Email: e-lartigau@o-lambret.fr.

2- and 5-year overall survival were respectively 39% and 13% and the logical conclusion was the necessity of treatment improvement trough precision and dose escalation studies.

More recently, the use of dosimetric CT scan offers the possibility to do multislice dosimetry and to switch from 2D to 3D. In 2005, a study [2] showed the advantage of 3D radiotherapy (3DRT) vs. 2DRT in terms of overall survival and local control. This study included 200 patients with stage I lung cancer treated by radiotherapy alone in two groups. The first group received 2DRT and the second group 3DRT. There were 115 patients in the 2DRT group, median age were 69 (range 44–88). 51% of patients presented T1N0 and 49% a T2N0, 47% had a squamous cell carcinoma and 53% a non-squamous histology. Median delivered dose was 64 Gy (40–74 Gy) and the median follow-up was 20 months (1–173 months). Eighty five patients in the second group were treated with 3DRT, they were 64% T1N0 and 36% T2N0 with 46% squamous cell carcinoma and 54% non-squamous histology. The median delivered dose was 66 Gy (45–90.3 Gy) and median follow-up was 19 months (3–77 months). The 2 years and 5 years overall survivals were respectively 47% and 10% for 2DRT and 68% and 36% for 3DRT (p=0.001). The 2 years and 5 years disease-specific survivals were respectively 62% and 29% for 2DRT and 83% and 68% for 3DRT (p=0.008). The 2 years and 5 years local-regional control were respectively 53% and 34% for 2DRT and 77% and 70% for 3DRT (p=0.0006). Different others studies shows the same kind of results, demonstrating the benefit of modern definition of treatment volumes and dose distribution. [3]

The Radiosurgery Concept

In parallel, since 1967 in Stockholm at the Karolinska Institut, Lars Leksell developed the concept of "Radiosurgery" with the Gammaknife. This high precision RT used more than 100 converging mini-beam, with a millimetric accuracy. This device was only intracranial as it was a mechanical accuracy with a stereotactic frame. Study after study, radiosurgery demonstrated a great efficacy to treat brain tumor, vascular lesions and functional disorders. General contraindications to radiosurgery includes today excessively large size of the target lesion (> 3 cm) or lesions too numerous for practical treatment. Radiosurgery outcome for brain tumor may not be evident until months after the treatment. Since radiosurgery does not remove the tumor, but results in a biological inactivation of the tumor, lack of growth of the lesion is normally considered to be treatment success. General indications for radiosurgery include many kinds of brain tumors, such as acoustic neuromas, germinomas, meningiomas, metastases, trigeminal neuralgia, arteriovenous malformations and skull base tumors. These results are limited to head treatment because of the necessity of a stereotactic frame.

Computerized Treatment and New Technologies

All the progresses demonstrated in the last 3 centuries have been made possible by the development of computer science, digital images and graphics. Computer graphics and digital image processing have evolved as two different technologies aimed at different application. Computer graphics were used usually for generating physical models, whereas digital images were used to capture X-rays. Merging these two technologies was called "visualization", and was applied for example to radiation treatment. These applications to radiation oncology conduce to 3D modeling and tracking capabilities. These tracking capabilities were applied to lock each treatment beam on a real time image, giving the possibility to remove the stereotactic frame and to start whole body stereotactic treatment. The most recent step has been the development of real time tracking capabilities to follow any target movement during irradiation through robotic SBRT.

Lung Tumor Treatment

Now with real time tracking capabilities of robotic SBRT, SBRT can be performed in any clinical situation with extreme precision. The technology of image guidance that the CyberKnife system can use is called the Synchrony system. The Synchrony software is used primarily for tumors that are in motion while being treated, such as lung tumors, with a combination of surgically placed internal fiducials and light emitting optical fibers (markers) placed on the patient skin. Since the tumor is moving continuously, permanent imaging would require prohibitive amounts of radiation to be delivered to the patients. The Synchrony system overcomes this by periodically taking images of the internal fiducials, and predicting their location at a future time using the motion of the markers that are located on the patient's skin. Then a computer algorithm creates a correlation model that represents how the internal fiducial markers are moving compared to the external markers. The Synchrony system is therefore continuously predicting the motion of the internal fiducials, and therefore the tumor, based on the motion of the markers. The advantage of the Synchrony system is that no assumptions about the regularity or reproducibility of the patient breathing have to be made. This concept allows a drastic increase of the dose in lung cancer.

Expectation

Brain and lung tumors are a "natural target" for cyberknife, but as there is no need for skeletal fixation, robotic SBRT can be applied to targets beyond the brain or the lung. The technology has been extensively used for stereotactic body radiotherapy, treating targets in many anatomic sites. Currently, clinical studies have been completed or are ongoing for common malignancies including tumors involving the spine, breast, pancreas, liver and prostate. In the first section we will see the natural history and the classification of lung cancer, then the indications of SBRT with Cyberknife. The second section will introduce the bio technical aspect with the radiobiology of large fraction, then a description of the system and the different tracking methods. Third section will present the results of Cyberknife treatment for small Peripheral tumours, central tumours, stage III tumors, reirradiation, lung metastasis and a review of toxicities.

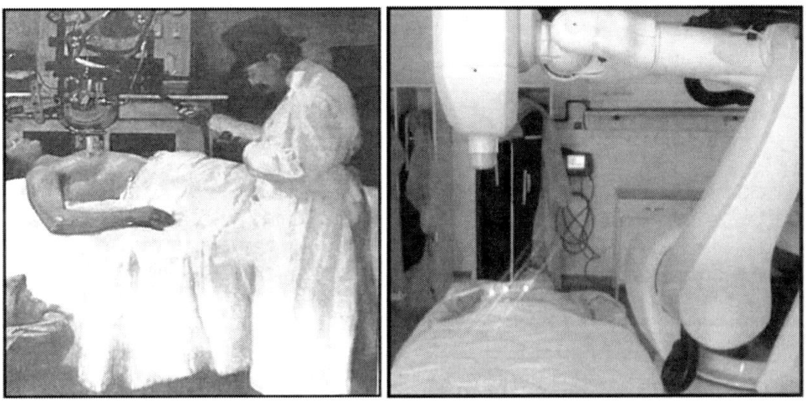

Figure 1. Robotic evolution of radiotherapy: Left, irradiation by Dr. Chicoto in 1907. Right. Robotic thoracic treatment in 2007.

References

[1] Sibley GS, Jamieson TA, Marks LB, Anscher MS, Prosnitz LR. Radiotherapy alone for medically inoperable stage I non-small-cell lung cancer: the Duke experience. *Int J Radiat Oncol Biol Phys*. 1998 Jan 1;40(1):149-54.

[2] Fang LC, Komaki R, Allen P, Guerrero T, Mohan R, Cox JD. Comparison of outcomes for patients with medically inoperable Stage I non-small-cell lung cancer treated with two-dimensional vs. three-dimensional radiotherapy. *Int J Radiat Oncol Biol Phys*. 2006 Sep 1;66(1):108-16.

[3] Hayman JA, Martel MK, Ten Haken RK, Normolle DP, Todd RF 3rd, Littles JF, Sullivan MA, Possert PW, Turrisi AT, Lichter AS. Dose escalation in non-small-cell lung cancer using three-dimensional conformal radiation therapy: update of a phase I trial. *J Clin Oncol*. 2001 Jan 1;19(1):127-36.

In: The Revolution of Robotic …
Editor: Pierre-Yves Bondiau
ISBN: 978-1-62808-718-5

Chapter 2

History of Lung Cancer and Its Treatment

Jérôme Mouroux*
Department of Thoracic Surgery, Hôpital Pasteur,
Centre Hospitalier Universitaire de Nice, France
University of Nice Sophia-Antipolis, Nice, France

Abstract

In 1878, lung cancer represented only 1% of all cancers in autopsy series. Despite its rarity, clinical descriptions of the disease multiplied beginning from the mid-19th century. However, the diagnosis was rarely made with certainty, because it was easy to confuse the cancer with tuberculosis. The disease was always fatal. At the beginning of the 20th century, the role of tobacco was mentioned and the incidence increased during World War I. Decisive advances resulted from the advent of radiology and development of bronchoscopy. Many surgeons considered treating the disease by lobectomy or pneumonectomy and they seemed at this period to be the standard treatment. Then, thanks to this classification, surgical results could be put in relation to the histologic type, and thus it appeared that surgery was not beneficial for small-cell cancer. With the introduction of mediastinoscopy, it became possible to

* Email: mouroux.j@chu-nice.fr.

explore the mediastinal lymph node sites. This chapter will present the history of lung cancer and the evolution of its surgical treatment.

Introduction

Bronchopulmonary cancer (BPC) is a major public health problem in all Western countries, with more than 30,000 new cases each year in France and more than 150,000 in the United States. Interest in this disease goes back to the 19th century. Lung cancer was first likened to a form of tuberculosis. Gaspard Laurent Bayle described "cancerous phthisis" as the most aggressive form in 1810. In 1819, Laennec isolated lung cancer and distinguished it from phthisis as a separate entity [1]. However, cases were rare and its incidence seemed very low. In 1878, lung cancer represented only 1% of all cancers seen on autopsy at the Pathology Institute of the University of Dresden [2]. In 1910, it represented 10% of all cancers. Onuigbo wrote on the clinical knowledge accumulated about the disease during this period including the description of the clinical manifestations and, in particular, the signs of compression described by Stokes in 1842, as well as the possibility of brain metastases reported by Cockle in 1868. Also at this time, the modes of lymphatic and blood-born dissemination of the disease were already described, and the first histological classification was established [3]. Unfortunately, the diagnosis was rarely made definitively during the life of the patient. In 1860, the great pathologist Rudolf Virchow recognized that, even at autopsy, it was possible to confuse cancer and tuberculosis. The disease was always fatal, because there was no specific treatment. In 1912, Adler published a book, *Primary Malignant Growths of the Lungs and Bronchi*, where he reported all known cases published in the world literature; 314 cases [4].

Around the end of the 19th century and the beginning of the 20th century, epidemiological studies established the connection between cancer and environmental causes of lung disease. Thus, cases of lung cancer in German miners from Schneeberg were recognized [2]. At the beginning of the 20th century, the role of cigarettes was mentioned as a potential cause of lung cancer. Beginning with the First World War, smoking increased, and the incidence of the disease increased considerably along with it. It would take the work of Doll and Hill in England in 1952 and the conclusions of the Study Group on Smoking and Health in 1957 for the role of smoking to be definitively established [5,6]. Subsequently, other work would confirm this finding and also name numerous other responsible factors, including occupational hazards [7]

Decisive advances in the diagnosis of the disease came with the discovery of radiology by Roentgen in 1895 and the development of bronchoscopy by Killian in 1897. Many surgeons, in Europe as well as in the United States, considered treating the disease by lobectomy or pneumonectomy. While these resection techniques were developed through numerous studies on animals, the essential difficulty lay in the fact that opening the thorax often caused a fatal lung collapse. Consequently, the procedures had to be carried out in several stages, and if the patient survived, it was at the cost of several weeks or months of hospitalization. To avoid this collapse, Sauerbruch created the first negative pressure chamber [8]. The work of Meltzer and Auer opened the era of modern thoracic surgery by creating anesthesia with tracheal intubation [9]. Thereafter, lung resection would develop mainly for infectious lesions such as tuberculosis or bronchiectases. In 1933, the first successful one-stage pneumonectomy for cancer was carried out by Evarts Graham in St Louis. It was performed on a 48-year-old physician, on April 5, 1933 [10]. The tumor was a squamous-cell carcinoma of the left lower lobe (afterwards classified T2N1). The patient lived until 1963 [11].

Very quickly, after this success, pneumonectomy became the standard therapeutic procedure for early stage lung cancer, because it could be quickly performed and appeared as an appropriate intervention for the disease. Graham established the contraindications for the procedure:

1. Presence of bloody pleural effusion
2. Phrenic paralysis
3. Paralysis of the left vocal cord
4. Severe chest pain, indicating an involvement of the intercostal nerves or brachial plexus
5. Evidence of involvement of the trachea
6. Presence of distant metastases.

The technique then consisted of a mass ligation, and concern for the management of the pleural space led to performing a thoracoplasty with rib resection shortly after the pneumonectomy. At the end of the 1930s and beginning of the 1940s, techniques for effective ligature of the vessels were developed, which were already proposed by Davies in 1912, to replace the mass ligature of the pedicle [12]. Also, at the bronchial level, the healing process was better understood and bronchial closure procedures were developed [13]. Despite these technological advances, mortality remained high. In 1939, Overholt, in a review of the literature, reported mortality for pneumonectomy for cancer at 65%, and 33.3% in his personal experience [14]. Some groups – such as those of Churchill, Belsey, and Overholt – were already proposing, where possible, lobectomy as the resection of choice [15]. During the next 10 years, debates focused on the best surgical approach to BPC: lobectomy vs. pneumonectomy [16]. The work of Shimkin, comparing the results of the two American thoracic surgeons, Overholt and Ochsner, helped clarify the debate [17]. Survival was similar between the procedures, but the operative morbidity was higher after pneumonectomy. As a result, lobectomy became the procedure of choice for BPC. Pneumonectomy was reserved for cases in which it was the only technique that could guarantee a complete resection.

Surgery seemed at this period to be the standard treatment, but two major problems were appearing: patient selection with potentially resectable tumors and a high number of serious, often fatal, postoperative septic complications.

The Pivotal Years: 1950–1980

It was in 1957 that Robbins introduced the first histological classification consisting of three main groups: squamous-cell carcinoma, adenocarcinoma, and undifferentiated cancer [18]. Subsequently, this classification would be refined under the aegis of the World Health Organization, arriving at the 4th classification, which is currently used [19]. Thanks to this classification, surgical results could be put into perspective according to the histologic type, and thus it appeared that surgery was not beneficial for small-cell carcinoma. In 1966, the Medical Research Council showed that small-cell carcinoma was not treatable surgically [20].

During this period, therapists became aware of the importance of an appropriate assessment of BPC before proposing therapy. In fact, in the 1960s, half of the patients were deemed inoperable, and for half of the operable patients, the tumor was unresectable. Exploratory thoracotomy rates ranged from 40% to 60% [16,21]. The decline of surgery was due either to the technical impossibility of resecting the tumor or to the significance of the mediastinal lymph node extension. At that time, cancers were detected and evaluated by x-ray, then later by CT. They were the only tools available for establishing the staging of the disease.

With the introduction of mediastinoscopy by Carlens in 1959, it became possible to explore the mediastinal lymph node sites [22]. Other variants appeared later: anterior mediastinotomy and mediastinopleuroscopy [23]. These procedures would establish the true lymph node status of the tumor, and thus improving the selection of operable patients. In the late 1970s, with the development of computed tomography (CT) and then magnetic resonance imaging (MRI) a few years later, clinicians were better able to clarify the characteristics of the tumor: its primary site, its size, and its relationship with the mediastinum and chest wall [24,25]. Lymph node involvement was detected, but mediastinoscopy was indispensable in order to histologically confirm nodal involvement. At the end of the 1980s, the concomitant use of CT, in some cases MRI, and if necessary mediastinoscopy, allowed the rate of exploratory thoracotomies to drop below the bar of 15%, and even 10% for certain teams [26,27].

In parallel with the development of the means of evaluation, a method of classifying tumors according to their level of extension was created. This method was due to the work of Denoix in 1946, and has been applied to all cancers [28]. Its principle was based on the classification of tumors according to the size and the local extension of the primary tumor (T), its lymphatic spread (N), and the presence of metastases (M). This classification established progressive stages (I-IV) to better understand prognosis, compare studies, and develop therapeutic strategies. In 1974, the first TNM classification dedicated to BPC was published [29]. This classification would be regularly improved, and currently the 7th edition is in place [30,31]. Mapping of the lymph nodes would be subsequently established, giving each lymph node site a specific number from 2 to 9 for the mediastinal lymph nodes, and 10 to 14 for the pulmonary lymph nodes [32].

During this period, progress was significant in the development of surgery for BPC. Creation of selective intubation, introduced by Carlens as early as 1949, improved the techniques of anesthesia, analgesia, and recovery [33]; and also the use of antibiotics and improvement of surgical instruments, especially the advent of surgical staplers, were witnessed during this period. The effect of these advances is apparent in the results of postoperative mortality as reported by Wilkins et al., who studied the changes in mortality after pneumonectomy at the Massachusetts General Hospital over 4 decades. Postoperative mortality went from 55.6% between 1934 and 1940, to 14.7% between 1941 and 1950, to 13.8% between 1951 and 1960, and to 11.1% between 1961 and 1970 [34].

Then, history repeated itself. A new debate on surgery emerged among surgeons, this time between supporters of lobectomy as the standard procedure and proponents of sublobar resections (segmentectomy). In the early 70s, Jensik et al., reported a clinical trial concerning segmentectomies performed for tumors whose size was at maximum 3–4 cm. The series was divided into three groups: group 1 contained previously operated patients (17 patients), group 2 was of palliative indications (36 patients), and group 3 had curative indications (69 patients) [35]. In this last group of 69 patients treated with curative intent, the authors reported 5 year survival at 56.4%. Postoperative mortality reported for all 123 patients was 4.8%.

The randomized trial conducted by the Lung Study Group demonstrated that the risk of recurrence was multiplied by 3 in the case of sublobar resection. Consequently, the primacy of lobectomy combined with lymphadenectomy had prevailed [36]. The Guidelines currently still recommend lobectomy as the standard procedure for BPC. The more limited resections are allowed for patients with limited cardio-respiratory function. In those cases, it's a surgical compromise and the patients are theoretically exposed to risk of recurrence.

Despite better disease staging, better patient selection, and surgical progress, the poor prognosis of the disease would soon encourage clinicians to propose additional treatments to surgery. Thus, the first randomized studies of BPC treatment began. Preoperative radiotherapy for BPC, a popular option in the 1960s, was then revealed to be without benefit [37]. The first trial of adjuvant therapy used Bacille Calmette Guérin (BCG) after complete resection of stage I cancer. The results showed no benefit compared with the control group [38]. From that time on, many cytotoxic products would be tested on non-small-cell BPC. Among the more than 50 drugs tested until the beginning of the 1980s, a greater than 15% response rate was shown for the following products: cisplatin, vindesine, vinblastine, mitomycin, and ifosfamide. Studies comparing these drugs to immunotherapy then showed superior efficacy. It was at this time that trials were initiated combining surgery with neoadjuvant or adjuvant treatment, with, in some trials, the use of radiation therapy.

1990s to the Present Day

The previous decades have resulted in major progress in treatment at all levels of BPC: the pre-therapeutic evaluation of the disease being more precise, yielding improved surgical results.. Postoperative mortality rates were less than 3% for lobectomy, which became the standard procedure (60% to 70% of procedures performed). Postoperative mortality for pneumonectomy fell below 10% [39-40]. Chemotherapy for inoperable forms showed its superiority to only palliative treatment, and to a certain extent, progress in the median survival of patients [41]. However, long-term results remained disappointing. In early 1990s, the 5 year survival rate for non-small-cell lung cancer, all stages combined, ranged between 13% and 15% [42]. This observation would stimulate interest in all areas of research, clinical as well as fundamental and translational. The last 20 years have been rich in progress.

Progress in the Evaluation of the Disease

The improvement in determination of the tumor stage is related to the development of metabolic imaging and minimally invasive medico-surgical procedures. Positron emission tomography (PET), based on the biological activity of neoplastic cells, allows better detection of lymph node involvement and/or remote metastases. Even though this examination is not infallible, several studies have shown that PET scans can avoid 20% of unnecessary thoracotomies [43-44].

At the same time, minimally invasive procedures have been introduced. Esophageal and bronchial echo-endoscopy for mediastinal and hilar lymph node biopsy, videomediastinoscopy to explore the mediastinum more safely and efficiently, and videothoracoscopy (VT) to explore the pleural cavity and lymph node sites not accessible by videomediastinoscopy have found use [45-48]. All these means helped to better elucidate the pretreatment staging of the tumor (cTNM) thus further reducing the number of exploratory thoracotomies (less than 3%). This also led to better selection of an appropriate treatment strategy by multidisciplinary clinical case discussion, an essential prerequisite to better treatment [49].

Advances in Histopathology and Molecular Biology

The work of Nokuchi et al., in 1995, observing differences in adenocarcinoma prognosis, would lead to reclassifying adenocarcinomas into subtypes [50], a classification which would be validated by the international community [51]. These years were marked by the discovery of various genetic and molecular modifications, which would open the way to targeted therapies. The last decade witnessed the significant success of personalized cancer treatment. This change of the therapeutic paradigm has led to considerable improvements in the clinical course of patients with tumors of molecularly defined subsets [52].

Treatment Progress

Surgery would see new technological progress, beginning in 1990, with the use of VT for diagnosis and then treatment, allowing precise lung resections. This practice is developing continuously for specific indications [53]. At present, almost 25% of resections are performed by VT in some centers. There is progress also in the type of pulmonary resections in paradoxically opposite directions. On the one hand, larger and safer resections, extending to the chest wall, spine, or even the mediastinal vessels [54,55], and on the other, parenchyma-sparing surgery reappearing. This latter approach, adopted by Jensik in the early 1970s, would resurface [35]. This development was due in large part to the discovery of small-size nodular lesions by increasingly frequent use of CT examinations and their precision, and also, to some extent, screening programs. The concept of parenchymal sparing would be taken up again as early as the mid-1990s by Read et al., [56]. These authors reported comparable survival in patients operated on for T1N0 tumors with lobectomy or segmentectomy. They reported survival as a function of the difference in tumor size, being either larger or smaller than 2 cm. They introduced the concept of tumor size correlating to parenchymal sparing. In 1997, Padilla et al., showed that survival of patients differed significantly, depending on whether the size of the tumor was less than 1 cm, between 1 cm and 2 cm, or greater than 2 cm. The 5-year survival rates were respectively 90%, 86.1%, and 65.4% [57]. The Japanese school showed the benefits of atypical resections for tumors smaller than 2 cm with a ground glass appearance, combined with a more or less significant solid component [58]. Okada et al., compared the survival of patients treated by lobectomy vs. segmentectomy for T1N0 cancers; survival was 87.1% and 87.7% respectively, without significant difference [59]. Sawabata et al., showed that there was no residual tumor when the safety margin was greater than the largest dimension of the tumor. These important aspects had to be known before deciding to carry out a sublobar resection [60]. At present, sublobar resection with a safety margin of at least 2 cm, with intraoperative analysis of the margins combined with lymph node dissection, may be proposed for lesions less than 2 cm [61]. On the other hand, inoperable patients may also benefit from technological progress due to the development of CyberKnife®

robotic stereotactic radiotherapy (Accuray Incorporated, Sunnyvale, CA) and/or radiofrequency ablation, with encouraging results [62-64].

Alongside these local treatments, systemic treatments have progressed. Several so-called "third generation" drugs such as vinorelbine, paclitaxel, docetaxel, gemcitabine, irinotecan, topotecan, and pemetrexed have shown activity.. Phase II trials with these new drugs have shown 20% to 30% response rates. The majority of phase III trials, comparing these products as monotherapy versus palliative care, have shown a benefit in terms of survival, and for some, in quality of life. Comparison of these active monotherapies with classic combinations used during the late 1980s (cisplatin + vindesine or etoposide) have shown identical survival, with a reduction in toxicity. In parallel with the development of new drugs, the results of therapeutic trials initiated in the late 1980s and early 1990s would come to reinforce the concept of multimodal treatment, especially in combination with surgery. This is why adjuvant chemotherapy is recommended, starting from stage II surgery, due to a beneficial effect on patient survival [65,66]. Similarly, chemotherapy and/or chemoradiotherapy induction treatments in locally advanced forms are now accepted [67,68].

In order to have optimal treatment of this increasingly complex disease, guidelines for good practices have been published at the national level. In addition, clinical case discussion (CCD) have been established, so that the best treatment decisions can be made [49]. Alongside these “technical” concerns, health authorities are urging all practitioners and institutions to initiate treatment programs to accommodate and involve the patient and his or her family and loved ones throughout the course of the treatment.

It has been 100 years since the first pneumonectomy was performed. Progress since then has been constant in all areas; diagnosis, staging, treatment modalities, and therapeutic strategies. Unfortunately, current results are not at a level making justice to the efforts made by the medical community. This disappointing fact is due in large part to the fact that the disease is still too often diagnosed at an advanced stage. Anti-smoking measures represent a major focus in reducing the incidence of the disease. Hope for improving treatment outcomes lies in screening for early diagnosis, but also in helping patients at risk of recurrence. Techniques currently being developed to recognize circulating cancer cells in the blood may be the key to screening in future years [69].

References

[1] Laënnec RTH : A treatise on the disease Chest, in which they are described according to their anatomical characters, and their diagnosis established on a new principe by means of acoustic instruments, translated by Jhon Forbes, MD Philadelphia, James Webster, 1823.

[2] Witschi H : A short history of lung Cancer. *Toxicol. Sci.* 2001; 64:4-6.

[3] Onuigbo W.I.B: Lung cancer in the nineteenth century. *Med. Hist.* 1959; 3:69-77.

[4] Spiro G, Silvestri GA. One hundred years of lung cancer. *Am. J. Respir. Crit. Care Med.* 2005; 172: 523-529.

[5] Doll R, Hill AB. A study of the aetiology of carcinoma of the lung. *Br. Med. J.* 1952; 2: 1271-86.

[6] Smoking ε Health Joint Report of the study Group on smoking and Health. *Science* 1957; 125: 1129-1133.

[7] Cornfield J; Haenszel W, Hammond EC, Lilienfeld AM, Shimkin MB, Wynder EL; Smoking and lung cancer: recent evidence and a discussion of some questions. *Int. J. Epidemil.* 2009; 38: 1175-1190.

[8] Sauerbruch F. Zur pathologie des offenen pneumothorax und die grundlagen meines verfahrens zu seiner ausschaltung, *Mitteilgen aus den Grenzgebieten der Medizin und Chirurgie* 1904; 13: 81-90.

[9] Meltzer SJ, Auer J. Continuous respirations without respiratory movements. *J. Exp. Med.* 1909; 11: 622-625.

[10] Graham E A : Primary carcinoma of the lung or bronchus. *Ann. Surg.* 1936; 103:1-12.

[11] Stanley C.F. A history of pneumonectomy. *Chest Surg. Clin. North Am.* 1999; 9:267-290.

[12] Davies HM. Recent advances in the surgery of the lung and pleura. *Br. J. Surg.* 1913; 1: 228-58.

[13] Rienhoff WF, Gannon J, Sherman I. Closure of the bronchus following total pneumonectomy. Experimental and clinical observations. *Ann. Surg.* 1942; 116: 481-531.

[14] Overholt R. Pneumonectomy for malignant and suppurative disease of the lung *J. Thorac. Cardiovasc. Surg.* 1939; 9 : 7-13.

[15] Fry WA. Chirurgie thoracique : historique et comparaison des développements en Europe et en Amérique du nord. *Rev. Mal. Respir* 2004 ; 21 : 369-71.

[16] Edwards AT. Carcinoma of the bronchus. *Thorax* 1946; 1: 1-25.

[17] Shimkin MB, Connelly BS, Marcus BS, Cutler SJ, Pneumonectomy and lobectomy in bronchogenic carcinoma. A comparison of end results of the Overholt and Ochsner Clinics. *J. Thorac. Cardiovasc. Surg.* 1962; 44:503-519.

[18] Robbins SL. Textbook of Pathology. Philadelphia, WB Saunders, 1957, pp 673-376.

[19] Travis WD, Brambilla E, Muller-Hermelink HK, Harris CC (Eds) World Heath Organisation. Classification of tumours. Pathology and Genetics of tumours of the lung, Pleura, Thymus and Heart. IARC Press: Lyon 2004.

[20] Medical Research Council: Comparative trial of surgery and radiotherapy for the primary treatment of small-celled or oat-celled carcinoma oft he bronchus. *Lancet* 1966; 2:979-986.

[21] Van den Bosch JMM, Gelissen HJ, Wagenar SS. Exploratory thoracotomy in bronchial carcinoma. *J. Thorac. Cardiovasc. Surg.* 1983; 85:733-737.

[22] Carlens E Mediastinoscopy : A method for inspection and tissue biopsy in the superior mediastinum. *Disease of the chest* 1959; 36:343-352.

[23] Deslauriers J, Beaulieu M, Dufour C, Michaud P, Despres JP, Lemieux M Mediastinoscopy : a new approach to the diagnosis of intrathoracic diseases.. *Ann. Thorac. Surg.* 1976, 22 :265-9.

[24] Ferguson MK, Mac Mahon H, Little A.G, Golomb H.M, Hoffman P.C, Skinner D.B. Regional accuracy of computed tomography of the mediastinum in the staging of the lung cancer. *J. Thorac. Cardiovasc. Surg.* 1986; 91: 71-77.

[25] Martini N, Heelan R, Wescott J, Bains M.S, Mc Cormack P, Caravelli J, Watson R, Zaman M. Comparative merits of conventional computed tomographic and magnetic resonance imaging in assessing mediastinal involvement in surgically comfirmed lung carcinoma. *J. Thorac. Cardiovasc. Surg.* 1985; 90: 639-648.

[26] Morand G, Roeslin N. La thoracotomie exploratrice de nécessité dans la chirurgie du cancer bronchique. *Ann. Chir.* 1990 ; 44 :133-137.

[27] Couraud L, Laurent F, Velly JF, Dorcier J, Zanotti L, Martigne C, Drouillard J. Apport respectif TDM et IRM au diagnostic d'opérabilité des cancers bronchiques. Bilan d'une confrontation TDM-IRM-Thoracotomie dans 111 cas. *Ann. Chir.* 1990 ; 44 :649-654.

[28] Denoix PF. Enquête permanente dans les centres anticancéreux. *Bull Inst. Nat. Hyg.* 1946, 1 : 70-75.

[29] Mountain CF, Carr DT, Anderson WAD : A system for the clinical staging of the lung cancer. *Am. J. of Roentgenol., Radium Ther. Nucl. Med* 1974;120:130-138.

[30] Mountain CF. Revision in the international system for staging lung cancer. *Chest* 1997; 111: 1710-1717.

[31] Goldstraw P, Crowley JJ. The International Association for the Study of Lung Cancer International Project on lung cancer. *J. Thorac. Oncol.* 2006; 1: 281-286.

[32] Mountain CF, Dresler CM Regional Lymph node classification for lung cancer staging *Chest* 1997 ; 111 : 1718-1723.

[33] Carlens E: A new flexible double-lumen catheter for bronchospirometry. *J. Thorac. Surg.* 1949 ; 18 :742-746.

[34] Wilkins EW, Scannel JG, Craver JG. Four decades of experiences with resections for bronchogenic carcinoma at the Massachusetts Hospital. *J. Thorac. Cardiovasc. Surg.* 1978; 76: 364-368.

[35] Jensik RJ, Penfield Faber L, Milloy FJ, Monson DO. Segmental resection for lung cancer. A fifteen-year experience. *J. Thorac. Cardiovasc. Surg.* 1974; 66: 563-572.

[36] Ginsberg RJ, Rubinstein LV Randomized trial of lobectomy versus limited resection for T1 N0 non-small cell lung cancer. *Ann. Thorac. Surg.* 1995; 60: 615-23.

[37] Warram J. Preoperative irradiation of cancer of the lung. Final report of a therapeutic trial. A collaborative study. *Cancer* 1975 ; 36 : 914-925.

[38] Holmes EC. Surgical results and surgical adjuvant therapy for lung cancer. *Am. J. Surg.* 1982; 143: 691-693.

[39] Ginsberg RJ, Hill LD, Eagan RT, Thomas P, Mountain CF, Deslauriers J, Fry WA, Butz RO, Goldberg M Waters PF, Jones DP, Pairolero P, Rubinstein L, Pearson G. Modern thirty-day operative mortality for surgical resections in the lung cancer. *J. Thorac. Cardiovasc. Sur.* 1983; 86:654-658.

[40] Patel RL, Townsend ER, Fountain SW. Elective pneumonectomy: factors associated with morbidity and operative Mortality. *Ann. Thorac. Surg.* 1992; 54: 84-88.

[41] Chemotherapy in non-small cell lung cancer:a meta-analysis using updated data on individual patients from 52 randomised clinical trials. Non-small Cell Lung Cancer Collaborative Group. *BMJ* 1995; 311: 899-909.

[42] Moro D, Nagy-Mignotte H, Bolla M, Colonna M, Brichon PY, Brambilla C, Schaerer R, Vrousos C. Evaluation de la survie et des

facteurs pronostics de 2000 cancers broncho-pulmonaires enregistrés en 10 ans dans une unité multidisciplinaire de cancérologie. *Bull du Cancer* 1997 ; 84 :155-161.

[43] Cerfolio RJ, Ojha B, Bryant A.S, Bass C.S Bartalucci A.A, Mountz J.M. The role of FDG-PET Scan in staging patients with nonsmall cell carcinoma. *Ann. Thor. Surg.* 2003; 76:861-866.

[44] Prevost A, Papathanassiou D, Jovenin N, Menéroux B, Cuif-Job A, Bruna-Muraille C, Domange-Testard A, Liehn J-C. Comparaison entre TEP-FDG et scanner dans le bilan d'extension du cancer broncho-pulmonaire, conséquences pour l'opérabilité chez 94 patients *Rev Pneumol Clin* 2009 ; 65 : 341-349.

[45] Kondo D, ImaizuniM, Abe T, Naruke T, Suemasu K ; Endoscopic ultrasound examination for mediastinal lymph node metastases of lung cancer. *Chest;* 1990: 586-593.

[46] Mentzer SJ, Swanson SJ, Decamps MM, Bueno R, Sugarbaker DJ. Mediastinoscopy, thoracoscopy and video-assisted thoracic surgery in the diagnosis and staging of lung cancer. *Chest* 1997; 112, 239S-241S.

[47] Mouroux J., Venissac N., Alifano. M.. Combined Video-assisted mediastinoscopy and video-assisted thoracoscopy in the management of lung cancer. *Ann. Thorac. Surg.* 2001; 72: 1698- 1704.

[48] Venissac, Alifano M, Mouroux J. Video-assisted mediastinoscopy : Experience from 240 consecutives cases. *Ann. Thorac. Surg.* 2003 ; 76 : 208-209.

[49] Leo F, Venissac N, Poudenx M, Otto J, Mouroux J.Multidisciplinary management of lung cancer: How to testits efficacy? *J. Thorac. Oncol.* 2007 ; 2 : 69-72.

[50] Noguchi M, Morikawa A, Kawasaki M, Matsuno Y, Yamada T, Hirohashi S, Kondo H, Shimosato Y. Small adenocarcinoma of the lung. Histologic characteristics and prognosis. *Cancer* 1995; 75: 2844-52.

[51] Travis WD, Brambilla E, NoguchiM et al., International association for the study of lung cancer /American thoracic society/European respiratory society international multidisciplinary classification of the lung adenocarcinoma. *J. Thorac. Oncol.* 2011; 6: 244-85.

[52] Silva S, Danson S. Targeted therapy and new anticancer drugs in advanced disease. *Thorac. Surg. Clin.* 2013; 23:411-419,

[53] Dewey TM, Mack MJ. Lung Cancer. Surgical approach and incisions. *Chest Surg. Clinof. North Am.* 2000; 10: 803-820.

[54] Deslauriers J, Tronc F, Fortin D. Management of tumors involving the chest wall including Pancoast Tumors and tumors invading the spine. *Thorac. Surg. Clin.* 2013; 23: 313-325.

[55] DiPerma C.A, Wood DE. Surgical management of T3 et T4 lung cancer. *Clin Cancer Res* 2005 ; 11(13suppl) :5038s5044s.

[56] Read RC, Yoder G, Schaeffer RC Survival after conservative resection for T1N0 M0 no-small cell lung cancer *Ann. Thorac. Surg.* 1990; 49: 391-400.

[57] Padilla J, Calvo V, Penalver JC, Sales G, Morcillo A. Surgical Results and prognostic factors in early non-small cell lung cancer. *Ann. Thorac. Surg.* 1997; 63: 324-326.

[58] Ikeda N, Maeda J, Yashima K, Tsuboi M, Kato H, Akada S, Okada S. A clinicopathological study of resected adenocarcinoma 2 cm or less in diameter. *Ann. Thorac. Surg.* 2004;78:1011-1016.

[59] Okada M, Yoshikawa K, Hatta T, Tsubota N. Is segmentectomy with lymph node assessement an alternative to lobectomy for non-small cell lung cancer of 2 cm or smaller. *Ann. Thorac. Surg.* 2001; 71: 956-960.

[60] Sawabata N, Ohta M, Matsumura A, Nakagawa K, Hirano H, Maeda H, Matsuda H, Optimal distance of malignant negative margin in excision of nonsmall cell lung cancer: A Multicenter prospective study. *Ann. Thorac. Surg.* 2004;77: 415-420.

[61] Okhada M. Radical sublobar resection for small-diameter lung cancers. *Thorac. Surg. Clin.* 2013; 23: 301-311.

[62] Blomgren H, Lax I, Näslund I, Svanström R; Stereotatic high dose fraction radiation therapy of extracranial tumors using an accelerator. Clinical experience of the first thirty-one patients. *Acta Oncol.* 1995; 34: 861-870.

[63] 63. Pennathur A, Luketich J.D, Heron DE, Abbas G, Burton S, Chen M, Gooding XE, Ozhasoglu C, Landreneau RJ, Christie NA. Stereotactic radiosurgery for the treatment of stage I non-small cell lung cancer in high-risk patients. *J. Thorac. Cardioovasc. Surg.* 2009; 137: 597-604.

[64] Choi J.Y, Kang S-G, Byun J.N Kim Y.S, Kim Y.C, Lee S.I. Radiofrequency ablation of the lung cancer: preliminary report. *Korean Radiol. Soc.* 2001; 45: 271-275.

[65] Cisplatin-based adjuvant chemotherapy in patients with completely resected Non-Small-Cell Cancer. The international Adjuvant Lung Cancer Trial Collaborative Group. *N. Engl. J. Med.* 2004; 350: 351-360.

[66] Pignon JP, Tribodet H, Scagliotti GV, Douillard J-Y, Sheperd F.A, Stephens RJ, Dunant A, Torri V, Rosell R, Seymour L, Spiro S.G,

Rolland E, Fossati R, Aubert D, Ding K, Waller D, Le Chevalier T. Lung Adjuvant Cisplatin Evaluation : A Pooled Analysis by the LACE Collaborative Group. *J. Clin. Oncol.* 2008; 26: 3552-3559.

[67] Tieu BH, Sanborn RE, Thomas CR. Neoadjuvant therapy for resecable non-small Cell lung cancer with mediastinal lymph node involvement. *Thorac. Surg. Clin.* 2008; 18: 403-415.

[68] Uy K.L, Darling G, Xu W, YI Q-L, De Perrot M, Pierre A.F, Waddell T.K Johnston M.R, Bezjak A, Shepperd F.A, Keshavjee S. Improved results of induction chemoradiation before surgical intervention for selected patients with stage IIIA-N2 non-small cell lung cancer. *J. Thorac. Cardiovasc. Surg.* 2007; 134: 188-93.

[69] Hofman V, Ilie M, Long E, Selva E, Bonnetaud C, Molina T, Venissac N, Mouroux J, Vielh P, Hofman P. Detection of circulating tumor cells as a prognostic factor in patients undergoing radical surgery for non-small-cell lung carcinoma: comparison of the efficacy of the Cellsearch Assay TM and the isolation by size of epithelial tumor cell method. *Int. J. Cancer* 2011; 129: 1651-1660.

In: The Revolution of Robotic …
Editor: Pierre-Yves Bondiau
ISBN: 978-1-62808-718-5

Chapter 3

Lung Cancer Classification

Philippe Giraud*
Université Paris Descartes, Service d'Oncologie Radiothérapie,
Hôpital Européen Georges Pompidou, Paris, France

Abstract

In 2009, the International Association for the Study of Lung Cancer (IASLC) proposed a new version of the TNM staging system. This report contains the recommendations of this committee for changes to the T, N, and M descriptors and the proposals for the new stage groupings. The work is based on analyses of the 67,725 cases of non-small cell lung cancer (NSCLC) treated by all modalities of care between 1990 and 2000. Data were derived from 46 sources in more than 19 countries. Related findings were validated internally by geographic area and type of database and were validated externally by the North American Surveillance, Epidemiology and End Results Registries (SEER). Modifications include new cutoffs for tumor size, with tumors > 7 cm moving from T2 to T3; reallocating the category given to additional pulmonary nodules in some locations; and reclassifying pleural effusion as an M stage. In addition, it is proposed that T2bN0M0 cases be moved from stage IB to stage IIA, T2aN1M0 cases from stage IIB to stage IIA, and T4 N0-1M0 case. Changes would improve the alignment of TNM stage with prognosis and, in certain subsets, with treatment.

* Email: Philippe.giraud@egp.aphp.fr.

Introduction

An essential step in the approach to a patient's cancer is to define the stage of the tumor. This need for definition has led to the development of universally accepted stage-classification systems for most tumors [1-4]. The stage classification systems are periodically reviewed and refined by The Union Internationale Contre le Cancer (UICC) and the American Joint Committee on Cancer (AJCC) [5]. The most recent version of the staging system for lung cancer was published in 2009 (7th edition) [6-12].

I. Methods

In order to create international databases, The International Association for the Study of Lung Cancer (IASLC) launched a worldwide Tumor, Node, Metastases (TNM) staging project in 1996 [1]. The TNM staging system for lung cancer dates back to an initial proposal by Clifton Mountain [2, 3]. The staging project collected data from multiple sources and sites around the globe [5-8]. The time frame that was used for data collection included all patients treated between the beginning of 1990 and the end of 2000. Cases were screened for adequate follow-up, histology, and baseline TNM staging. The total number of patients submitted to Cancer Research and Biostatistics was 100,869. Of this total, 81,015 met the following initial screening requirements: a new diagnosis (rather than a diagnosis of recurrent disease), small cell lung cancer (SCLC) or non–small cell lung cancer (NSCLC), adequate follow-up (for survival calculations), and a complete set of either clinical TNM (cTNM) or pathological TNM (pTNM) at baseline.

The study population that passed the initial screening criteria contained 67,725 cases of NSCLC and 13,290 cases of SCLC. The two groups were analyzed separately, but only NSCLC cases will be analyzed in this chapter. The geographic sources (by continent) of the 67,725 NSCLC patients were as follows: 40,059 from Europe, 12,178 from North America, 10,216 from Asia, and 5,272 from Australia. Among all these NSCLC patients, 95% of them were followed until death or at least 2 years; and 88%, until death or 5 years. The median follow-up for the 17,754 patients who were still alive at last contact was 5.3 years.

The recommendations for lung cancer classification were internally and externally validated. The internal validation approach was to compare results of interest among types of databases (consortium/surgical series vs. clinical trials vs. series/registries) and geographic regions (North America vs. Australasia vs. Europe) [5-8, 13]. For external validation, the selected NSCLC cases were those who were diagnosed from 1998 to the end of 2000 from the Surveillance, Epidemiology, and End Results Program (SEER) database [14].

II. Classification

The NSCLC stage classification is based on the TNM system (which is used for most cancers). The T descriptor defines the extent of the primary tumor, the N descriptor refers to the extent of the involvement of the regional lymph nodes, and the M descriptor represents the extent of the spread to distant sites. The TNM staging system is based solely on the anatomic extent of disease. In lung cancer, however, nodal staging depends on the location of involved nodes (as opposed to the number of nodes). The M descriptor defines the presence or absence of more distant metastatic disease.

The major determinant that was chosen for the development of the T, N, and M descriptor subgroups (and the stage groupings) was overall survival. This determinant was based on the best stage of the tumor (pathologic, if available; otherwise, clinical).

II.1. T Descriptor

Tumor size has a major impact [6, 8, 10, 15, 16]. The size threshold of 3 cm was confirmed as a significant censored point and retained to differentiate a T1 vs. a T2 tumor. In addition, significant censored points were identified at 2, 5, and 7 cm. Tumors > 7 cm had survival that tracked with other definitions of T3 (i.e., invasion or central location) and are therefore placed within that group. The additional 2 and 5 cm cut-points were addressed by the definition of subgroups of T1 (T1a and T1b) and T2 (T2a and T2b) (Table 1; Figures 1, 2) [10].

Patients with additional satellite nodules in the same lobe as the primary tumor had relatively good survival, similar to that of T3 patients, and therefore are classified as T3 (previously classified as T4). An ipsilateral nodule in a different lobe is, however, classified as T4 (previously classified as M1) (Table 1; Figures 3, 4).

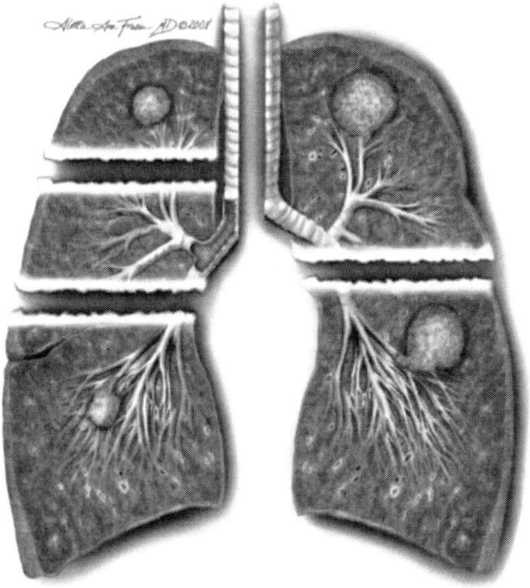

Figure 1. Graphic illustration of T1 (T1a on left, T1b on right). *Courtesy of La lettre du cancérologue, Edimark SAS.*

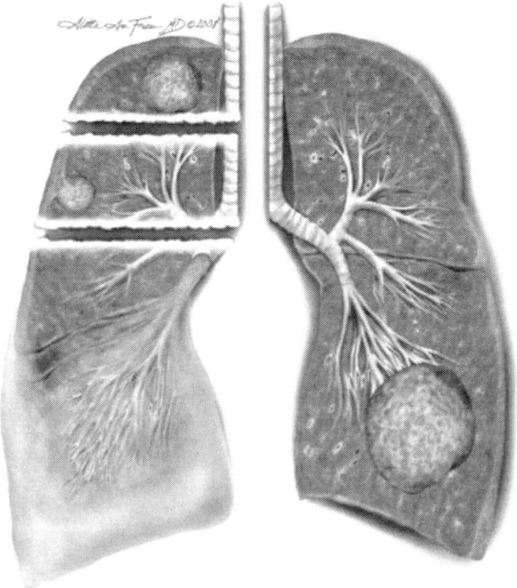

Figure 2. Graphic illustration of T2 (T2a on left, T2b on right). *Courtesy of La lettre du cancérologue, Edimark SAS.*

Table 1. Definitions for T, N, and M descriptors: T (primary tumor)

Descriptors	Definitions
TX	Primary tumor cannot be assessed
T0	No evidence of primary tumor
Tis	Carcinoma in situ
T1	Tumor ≤ 3 cm in the greatest dimension, surrounded by lung or visceral pleura, and not more proximal than the lobar bronchus (i.e., not in the main bronchus).
T1a	Tumor ≤ 2 cm in the greatest dimension
T1b	Tumor > 2 cm but ≤ 3 cm in the greatest dimension
T2	Tumor > 3 cm but ≤ 7 cm in the greatest dimension or tumor with any of the following features: invades visceral pleura, involves main bronchus ≥ 2 cm distal to the carina, has atelectasis/obstructive pneumonia extending to hilum but not involving the entire lung. T2 with these features are classified T2a if ≤ 5 cm.
T2a	Tumor > 3 cm but ≤ 5 cm in the greatest dimension
T2b	Tumor > 5 cm but ≤ 7 cm in the greatest dimension
T3	Tumor > 7 cm or directly invading chest wall, diaphragm, phrenic nerve, mediastinal pleura, or parietal pericardium; or tumor in the main bronchus < 2 cm distal to the carina or atelectasis/obstructive pneumonitis of entire lung or separate tumor nodule(s) in the same lobe.
T4	Tumor of any size with invasion of mediastinum, heart, great vessels, trachea, recurrent laryngeal nerve, esophagus, vertebral body, or carina; or separate tumor nodule(s) in a different ipsilateral lobe.

II.2. N Descriptor

Analysis of the prognostic influence of the N descriptor clearly supported the traditional categorizations of N0, N1, N2, and N3. Several nodal zones were defined: an upper zone (stations 1 to 4), an aortopulmonary zone (stations 5 and 6), a subcarinal zone (station 7), a lower zone (stations 8 and 9), a hilar zone (stations 10 and 11), and a peripheral zone (stations 12 to 14) (Figure 5) [4, 7, 12]. There was no difference in survival among patients with involvement of only peripheral N1 nodes or hilar N1 nodes or in the various N2 nodal stations.

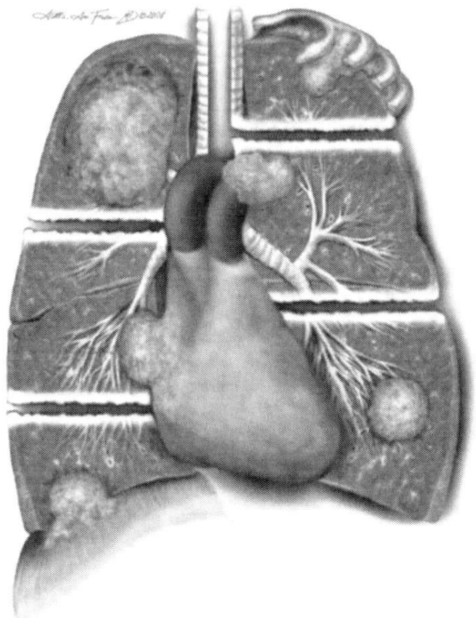

Figure 3. Graphic illustration of T3. Courtesy of La lettre du cancérologue, Edimark SAS.

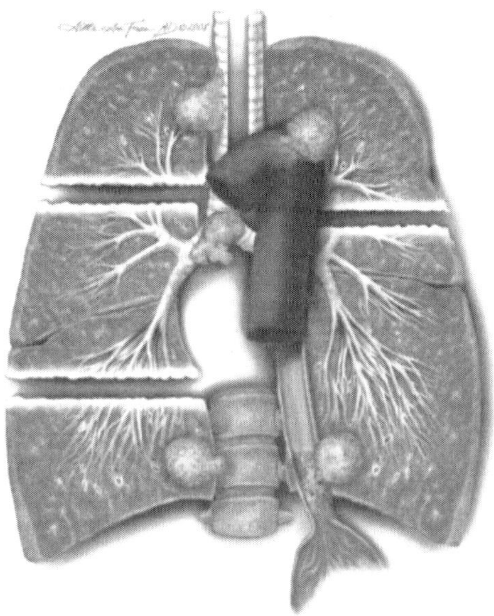

Figure 4. Graphic illustration of T4. Courtesy of La lettre du cancérologue, Edimark SAS.

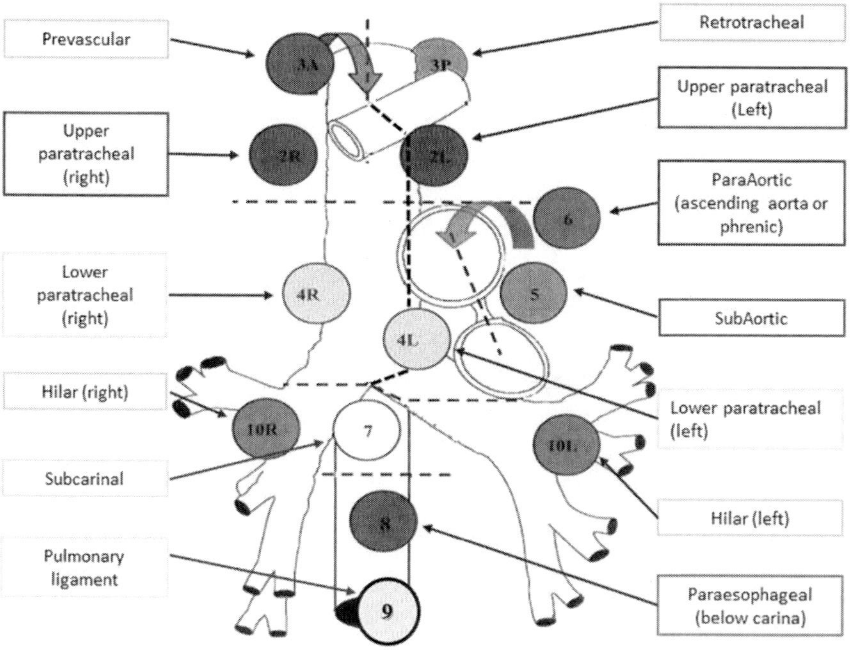

Figure 5. The lymph nodes map [11, 12].

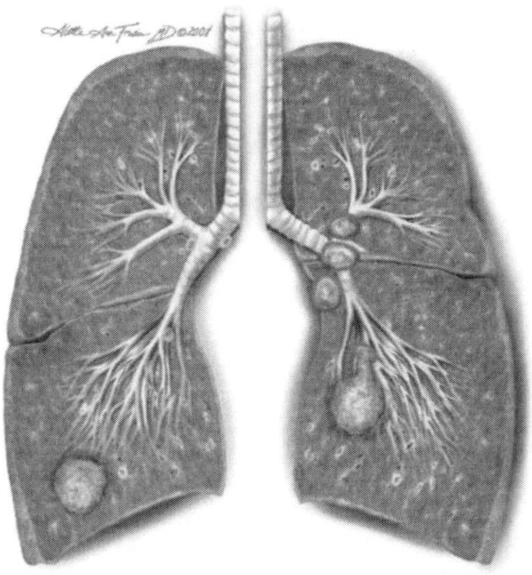

Figure 6. Graphic illustration of N0 on left and N1 on right. *Courtesy of La lettre du cancérologue, Edimark SAS.*

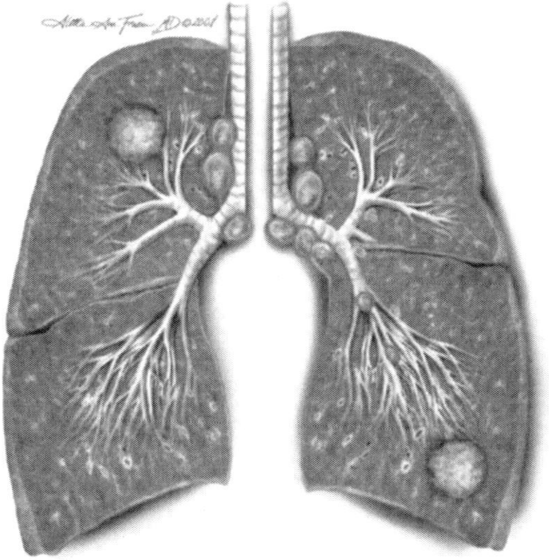

Figure 7. Graphic illustration of N2. Courtesy of La lettre du cancérologue, Edimark SAS.

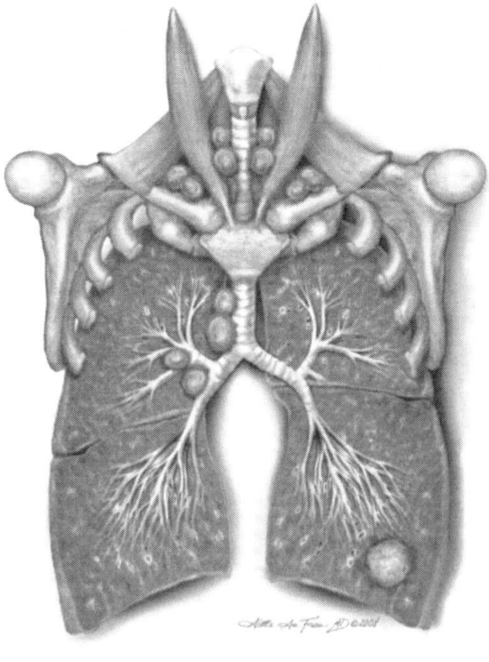

Figure 8. Graphic illustration of N3. Courtesy of La lettre du cancérologue, Edimark SAS.

Table 2. Definitions for T, N, and M descriptors: N (regional lymph nodes)

Descriptors	Definitions
NX	Regional lymph node(s) cannot be assessed
N0	No regional lymph node metastasis
N1	Metastasis in ipsilateral peribronchial and/or ipsilateral hilar lymph node(s) and intrapulmonary node(s), including involvement by direct extension
N2	Metastasis in ipsilateral mediastinal and/or subcarinal lymph node(s)
N3	Metastasis in contralateral mediastinal, contralateral hilar, ipsilateral or contralateral scalene, or supraclavicular lymph node(s)

Table 3. Definitions for T, N, and M descriptors: M (distant metastasis)

Descriptors	Definitions
MX	Distant metastasis cannot be assessed
M0	No distant metastasis
M1	Distant metastasis
M1a	Separate tumor nodule(s) in a contralateral lobe or tumor with pleural nodules or malignant pleural (or pericardial) effusion
M1b	Extrathoracic metastasis

Table 4. Definitions for T, N, and M Descriptors: Stage Groups

T / M	N0	N1	N2	N3
T1 T1a	IA	IIA	IIIA	IIIB
T1b	IA	IIA	IIIA	IIIB
T2 T2a	IB	IIA	IIIA	IIIB
T2b	IIA	IIB	IIIA	IIIB
T3	IIB	IIIA	IIIA	IIIB
T4	IIIA	IIIA	IIIB	IIIB
M1 M1a	IV	IV	IV	IV
M1b	IV	IV	IV	IV

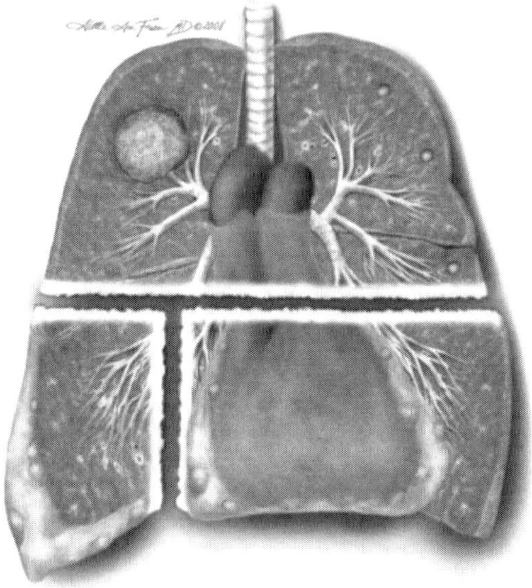

Figure 9. Graphic illustration of M1a. Courtesy of La lettre du cancérologue, Edimark SAS.

However, the number of involved nodal zones did appear to have a prognostic impact. Patients with single-zone N1 involvement had better survival than those with multizone N1 involvement (5-year survival rate, 48% vs. 35%, respectively; $p < 0.09$). Similarly, patients with single-zone N2 involvement had better survival than those with multizone N2 involvement (5-year survival rate, 34% vs. 20%, respectively; $p < 0.001$). In fact, the survival curves of patients with multizone N1 and single-zone N2 involvement could almost be superimposed (Table 2; Figures 6-8) [6, 7, 11].

II.3. M Descriptor

The committee that worked with the M descriptor considered patients that were traditionally classified as M0 or M1 (distant metastases), but it also considered patients with a malignant pleural effusion or additional tumor nodules in the lung. The M1a subgroup included patients with either pleural dissemination or contralateral pulmonary nodules and the M1b subgroup included patients with distant metastases (Table 3; Figures 9, 10) [6, 7, 9].

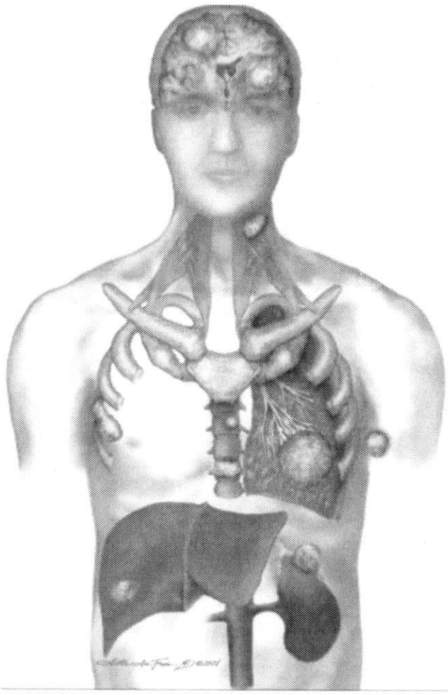

Figure 10. Graphic illustration of M1b. Courtesy of La lettre du cancérologue, Edimark SAS.

II.4. Stage Grouping

The IASLC International Staging Committee has defined stage groupings (Table 4) [6, 7].

III. Discussion

The IASLC system clearly meets the need for a common nomenclature. However, it should be keep in mind that the optimal treatment is defined by clinical trials, and eligibility for a particular treatment depends on multiple factors, including modality-related factors, patient-related factors (e.g., performance status or comorbidities), and tumor-related factors (e.g., histology, stage, or proximity to other organs). However, the IASLC's staging system provides a nomenclature to facilitate the discussion of one aspect of the applicability of clinical trial results to newly diagnosed patients [1, 2, 17].

The definitions of the TNM descriptors and their stage groups were determined primarily by the outcome measure of overall survival. This measure was chosen because the prognosis for anatomic categories of disease was the only outcome measure and method of patient characterization for which data exists for a large number of patients. The recommendations for the TNM descriptors and their stage groups were based on the findings of a large international database [4, 8, 18]. However, advances in imaging alter the stage assignment of a patient (stage migration), which affects the prognosis of all stage groups. Additionally, changing the methods of detection (e.g., CT or PET screening) can alter the spectrum of disease that is encountered [6, 19].

The most recent IASLC classification proposed changes that suggest the establishment of size cutoffs as well as the 3 cm limit that differentiates T1 and T2 tumors. Tumors that are defined as T1 but are also 2 cm in their greatest dimension should be designated T1a, whereas T1 tumors that are > 2 cm but < 3 cm in their greatest dimension should be designated T1b. Those tumors that fulfill the present definition of T2 but are < 5 cm in greatest dimension should become T2a, whereas those that are > 5 cm but < 7 cm in greatest dimension should become T2b. A tumor dimension of > 7 cm should become a T3 descriptor. Other proposed changes include that additional tumor nodules in the lobe of the primary lung become T3, nodules in other ipsilateral lobes become T4, and nodules in the contralateral lung remain classified as M1 disease.

The presence of a malignant pleural effusion, pleural dissemination, or pericardial disease would give a tumor an M descriptor. The M category would subdivide into M1a (which includes the new descriptors added to this category, i.e., cases with pleural nodules or malignant pleural or pericardial effusion and additional pulmonary nodules in the contralateral lung) and M1b (for those cases with other distant metastases). The proposed system better delineates the early-stage cases, where there are problems with overlap between IB and IIA. The distinction between clinical IIA and IIB would also be improved. Furthermore, moving the larger node-negative T2 tumors (T2b cases > 5 cm in their greatest dimension) and tumors that are > 7 cm in their greatest dimension (which would become T3) from stage IB into stage IIA and stage IIB, respectively, will clearly raise the question as to whether such cases should have adjuvant chemotherapy after complete resection. This question results from the fact that doubt still remains as to the value of adjuvant chemotherapy after complete resection for node-negative cases in stage IB [6, 12].

Conclusion

The new IASLC staging classification is a major advance. This extensive effort has allowed worldwide experiences with lung cancer to be brought together to create the IASLC's evidence-based staging classification. Improvements to this classification will require the prospective collection of more data (according to the data elements defined by global experiences) and thoughtful investigation of novel factors that can be used as biological data and may thus enhance our understanding.

Classifying tumors by their molecular biological characteristics may actually be complementary, or even more useful, than the IASLC clinical proposals. Unfortunately, however, there is only a rudimentary ability to predict tumor biology, and only a limited number of patients have biological data available. Clinical observation suggests that tumors may have 4 different types of biological behaviors, and each tumor can be primarily characterized by the following propensities: to spread to regional lymph nodes, to invade directly and locally, to develop additional foci of cancer within the lung, and to disseminate systemically [20].

References

[1] Goldstraw P. The International Staging Committee of the IASLC: its origins and purpose. *Lung Cancer* 2002;37:345–8.

[2] Mountain CF, Carr DT, Anderson WAD. A system for the clinical staging of lung cancer. *Am. J. Roentgenol. Radiat. Ther. Nucl. Med.* 1974; 120:130–8.

[3] Mountain CF. Staging classification of lung cancer. A critical evaluation. *Clin. Chest Med.* 2002;23:103–21.

[4] Sculier J-P, Chansky K, Crowley J, Van Meerbeeck J, Goldstraw P. The impact of additional prognostic factors on survival and their relationship with the anatomical extent of disease expressed by the 6th Edition of the TNM Classification of Malignant Tumors and the proposals for the 7th Edition. *J. Thorac. Oncol.* 2008;3:457–66.

[5] Goldstraw P, Crowley J. The International Association for the Study of Lung Cancer International Staging Project on Lung Cancer. *J. Thorac. Oncol.* 2006; 1:281–6.

[6] Detterbeck F, Boffa D, Tanoue L. The New Lung Cancer Staging System. *Chest* 2009;136; 260-71.

[7] Goldstraw P, Crowley J, Chansky K, Giroux D, Groome P, Rami-Porta R, Postmus P, Rusch V, Sobin L. The IASLC Lung Cancer Staging Project: Proposals for the Revision of the TNM Stage Groupings in the Forthcoming (Seventh) Edition of the TNM Classification of Malignant Tumours. *J. Thorac. Oncol.* 2007;2:706–14.

[8] Groome P, Bolejack V, Crowley J, Kennedy C, Krasnik M, Sobin L, Goldstraw P. The IASLC Lung Cancer Staging Project: Validation of the Proposals for Revision of the T, N, and M Descriptors and Consequent Stage Groupings in the Forthcoming (Seventh) Edition of the TNM Classification of Malignant Tumours. *J. Thorac. Oncol.* 2007;2: 694–705.

[9] Postmus P, Brambilla E, Chansky K, Crowley J, Goldstraw P, Patz E, Yokomise H. The IASLC Lung Cancer Staging Project: Proposals for Revision of the M Descriptors in the Forthcoming (Seventh) Edition of the TNM Classification of Lung Cancer. *J. Thorac. Oncol.* 2007;2:686–93.

[10] Rami-Porta R, Ball D, Crowley J, Giroux DJ, Jett J, Travis WD, Tsuboi M, Vallières E, Goldstraw P. The IASLC Lung Cancer Staging Project: proposals for revision of the T descriptors in the forthcoming (seventh) edition of the TNM classification of lung cancer. *J. Thorac. Oncol.* 2007; 2:593–602.

[11] Rusch VW, Crowley JJ, Goldstraw P, Goldstraw P, Im JG, Tsuboi M, Tsuchiya R, Vansteenkiste J. The IASLC Lung Cancer Staging Project: Proposals for revision of the N descriptors in the forthcoming (seventh) edition of the TNM Classification of Malignant Tumours. *J. Thorac. Oncol.* 2007;2:706–14.

[12] Rusch VW, Asamura H, Watanabe H, Giroux DJ, Rami-Porta R, Goldstraw P. The IASLC Lung Cancer Staging Project: a proposal for a new international lymph node map in the forthcoming 7th edition of the TNM Classification for Lung Cancer. *J. Thorac. Oncol.* 2009; 4:568–77.

[13] Naruke T, Tsuchiya R, Kondo H, Asamura H. Prognosis and survival after resection for bronchogenic carcinoma based on the 1997 TNM staging classification: the Japanese experience. *Ann. Thorac. Surg.* 2001;71:1759–64.

[14] Surveillance, Epidemiology, and End Results (SEER) Program (www.seer.cancer.gov) SEER*Stat Database: Incidence–SEER 13 Regs Public-Use, November 2004 Sub (1973–2002 varying), National Cancer.

[15] Cangir AK, Kutlay H, Akai M, Güngör A, Ozdemir N, Akay H. Prognostic value of tumor size in non-small cell lung cancer larger than five centimeters in diameter. *Lung Cancer* 2004;46:325–31.

[16] Lopez-Encuentra A, Duque-Medina JL, Rami-Porta R, de la Cámara AG, Ferrando P. Staging in lung cancer: is 3 cm a prognostic threshold in pathologic stage I non-small cell lung cancer? A multicenter study of 1,020 patients. *Chest* 2002;121:1515–20.

[17] Detterbeck FC, Tanoue LT, Boffa DJ. Anatomy, biology and concepts pertaining to the lung cancer stage classification. *J. Thorac. Oncol.* 2009; 4:437–43.

[18] Berghmans T, Lafitte JJ, Thiriaux J, VanHoutte P, Lecomte J, Efremidis A, Koumakis G, Giner V, Richez M, Corhay JL, Wackenier P, Lothaire P, Mommen P, Ninane V, Sculier JP. Survival is better predicted with a new classification of stage III unresectable non-small cell lung carcinoma treated by chemotherapy and radiotherapy. *Lung Cancer* 2004;45:339–48.

[19] Morgensztern D, Goodgame B, Baggstrom M, Gao F, Govindan R. The effect of FDG-PET on the stage distribution of non-small cell lung cancer. *J. Thorac. Oncol.* 2008; 3:135–9.

[20] Van der Sijp JR, van Meerbeeck JP, Maat AP, Zondervan PE, Sleddens HF, van Geel AN, Eggermont AM, Dinjens WN. Determination of the molecular relationship between multiple tumors within one patient is of clinical importance. *J. Clin. Oncol.* 2002;20:1105–14.

In: The Revolution of Robotic …
Editor: Pierre-Yves Bondiau
ISBN: 978-1-62808-718-5

Chapter 4

Indication of CyberKnife in Lung Cancer

Michel Poudenx [*,1,2] ***and Pierre-Yves Bondiau*** [†,2,3]
[1]Department of Medical Oncology,
Antoine-Lacassagne Cancer Center, Nice, France
[2]University of Nice Sophia-Antipolis, Nice, France
[3]Department of Radiation Oncology,
Antoine-Lacassagne Cancer Center, Nice, France

Abstract

Indications of SBRT are divided in two categories; intracranial treatment and extracranial treatment. For extracranial treatment, SBRT can be used for lung treatment. Stage I NSCLC if medically inoperable or if patient refuses open surgery can be treated with SBRT. In some cases it can be used for advanced stage NSCLC as a boost treatment. In cases of lung metastases: solitary or limited (2-5) multiple metastases if symptomatic or enlarging on serial imaging with a favorable survival profile.

* michel.poudenx@nice.unicancer.fr.
† pierre-yves.bondiau@nice.unicancer.fr.

Primitive Lung Tumors

Lung cancer is now the leading cause of cancer death for both men and women in different countries, and continues to have a very low five-year survival rate of less than 15% [any stage] [1]. About 75 % of patients with lung cancer will be diagnosed with Non Small Cell Lung Cancer (NSCLC), and 15-20 % with an early (stage I-II) disease. Therefore, in the next few years, the number of patients diagnosed with stage I-II NSCLC is expected to rise significantly due to use of screening with spiral CT scanning.

Currently, complete surgical resection remains the best hope for cure, consisting of either lobectomy or pneumonectomy, resulting in five-year survival rates of approximately 40-60% for T1-2 N0 NSCLC [1,2]. However, not all patients with lung cancer are candidates for surgical resection. This chapter will describe what kinds of patients are eligible for lung cancer SBRT. In most of the cases, there are patients that cannot benefit from surgical resection of the lung tumor.

These patients:

- present insufficient ventilation, heart failure comorbidity, diabetes, vascular disease and other comorbidities cons-indicating surgery.
- are not candidates for anesthesia.
- are not candidates for resection because of anatomical or physiological factors.
- do not want surgery.

For these patients, conventional radiotherapy is a possible option but this treatment is limited by the dose and toxicity to adjacent organs and local control rate is low. SBRT allows increasing the dose to the tumor without causing complications in fragile patients; it is a perfect alternative to surgery for these cases.

The first studies using SBRT in lung diseases were conducted in the years *2000 to 2005* mainly in Japan and the USA. [3-9]. Patients was a mix of early NSCLC (inoperable or who refused surgery) and lung metastasis. These studies did not differentiate central and peripheral tumors. Results were consistent for patients with a Biological Equivalent Dose (BED) > *85 Gy* and provide a local control rate range from 85% to *95%*.

The largest published series of SBRT for NSCLC is a retrospective multicentre Japanese study reported by Onishi [10]. Patients (n=257) had a inoperable stage I-II NSCLC or declined surgery. For stage I-II patients treated with SBRT, five years overall survival compares favorably with US and Japanese surgical series. Moreover, in another study [11], the same author reports the results of 87 stages I NSCLC patients treated with SBRT. Unlike the previous study, all patients were medically operable but refused surgery. With a median follow-up of 55 months, local control rates at 5 years were 72% and 62% respectively.

Results are summarized in table 1.

Table 1. Result of Japan and US series for surgery and SBRT

	SURGERY*		SBRT	
	USA [4]	**JAPAN [5]**	**All NSCLC pts [3]**	**Operable [2]**
Stage IA	61%	71%	72%	76%
Stage IB	40%	44%	66%	64%

* Lobectomy or Pneumonectomy.

SBRT is now a standard of care for stage I-II non operable patient. The first studies did not differentiate treatment and results based on the peripheral or central location of the tumors. A central location of the tumor, may theoretically result in increased side effects of radiotherapy because the proximity of organs at risk (great vessels, heart, esophagus, bronchial tree, spinal cord). A study of different fractionation separately of central and peripheral tumors seems of great importance in terms of safety and efficacy.

Stage I-II Peripheral Tumors

Peripheral Tumors are usually defined in most studies by a distance equal or greater than 2 cm relative to the proximal bronchial tree defined as the distal 2 cm of trachea, carina, and named major lobar bronchi up to their first bifurcation (Cf. Figure 1).

Despite the vast majority of peripheral tumors (> 70%) in the studies mentioned above, the results in terms of local control and survival were not always differentiated.

In the study from the University of Indiana [12], 70 patients (48 peripheral, 22 central) treated with SBRT, the local control rates at 3 years for the entire population was 88.1% and overall survival at 3 years of 42, 7%. There was no difference in median survival between the peripheral tumors (35.9 months) and proximal tumor (24.4 months) p = 0439.

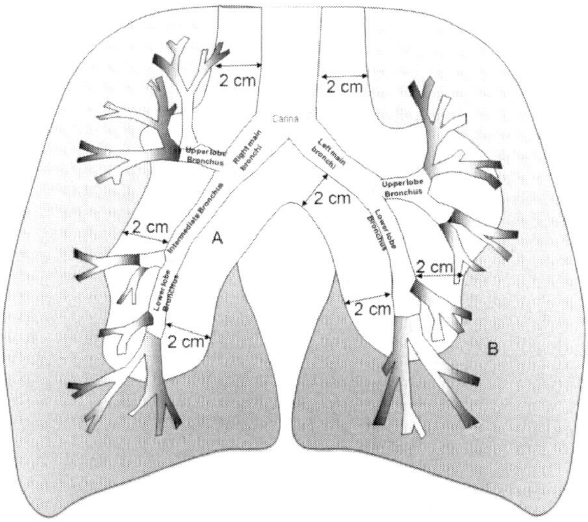

Figure 1. Central (A) or peripheral (B) tumor.

In the RTOG phase II multicenter study reported by Timmerman [13], 55 inoperable stage II NSCLC patients were treated by SBRT. All patients had a peripheral tumor <5 cm of diameter located more than 2 cm of the proximal bronchial tree. At a median follow-up of 34.4 months, the 3-year control rate was 97.6 % and the 3-year overall survival rate was 55.8%

Haasbeek and colleagues [14] did not find any difference in overall survival and local control rates by comparing a retrospective series of 445 patients with peripheral tumors and 63 patients with a central tumor location treated by stereotactic irradiation (3 year local control rate 90,2% vs. 92,6% respectively; p=0.9)

Van der Voort Van Zyp et al. [15], have treated 70 patients with NSCLC stage IA and IB and non-central tumor with CyberKnife. The 2-year local control was 96% for patients treated with 60 gy (BED =180 gy) compared to 78% for patients treated with a total dose of 45 Gy (BED = 112,5 gy) This study confirm the dose intensity efficacy.

Stage I-II Central Tumor

In the previously cited study by The Indiana University [12], local control and overall survival was similar between central and peripheral lesion but toxicity was more common on central tumors with a 27,3% grade 3-5 toxicity compare with 10,8% for peripheral tumors. These increases of toxicity have not been found in other studies. Senthi et al., [16] have recently reviewed studies reporting results of SBRT for centrally located tumors (primary NSCLC or metastatic lung tumor). Twenty publications were reviewed including 315 patients with early stage NSCLC. Results are summarized in table 2.

For these authors, tumor location (peripheral vs. central) did not impact overall survival and local control rates for central tumors were ≥ 85% when the prescribed biologically equivalent tumors dose was ≥ 100 grays. Interesting, grade 3-4 toxicities seems more frequently observed in central tumors but occurred in less than 9% of patients. Grade 5 lethal toxicities occurred in only 11 patients of this study including esophageal toxicities, bronchial toxicities (fistula, stenosis) and haemoptysis.

SBRT for central lung tumors is feasible for achieving high local control rates with limited toxicity. However, toxicity seems higher than peripheral lesions and prospective data to determine fractionation schedules and reliable normal organ constraints are needed. The RTOG 0813 trial is ongoing questioning this point.

SBRT Compare to Limited "Curative" Resection

Grills et al., [17] had compared in patients with a limited pulmonary reserve SBRT to wedge resection. One hundred twenty four NSCLC stage I-II N0 patients were studied (69 wedge, 58 SBRT). Patients in the radiotherapy group were medically inoperable at physician's discretion (95%) or refusal of surgery (5%). Characteristics of the patients showed a significant difference between the two groups for comorbidity and median age (Respectively SBRT versus Wedge; Charlson's score 4 vs. 3 p =0.01 and age 78 years vs. 74 years p = p=0.04). There was no difference in lung function (Forced Expiratory Volume 1.39 L vs. 1.31 L and Diffusing Capacity of Lung for Carbon Monoxide 12,1 mL/mn vs. 10,14 mL/mn).

Table 2. Survival and local control

Author (year)	BED_{10}	Overall survival	Cause-specific survival	Local control
Chang [26] (2008)	113	–		Crude rate 89%
Song [36] (2009)	106	50% at 2 years	–	89% at 2 years
Milano [27] (2009)	100	72% at 2 years	–	73% at 2 years
Fakiris [24] (2009)	180	Median 24 months	–	–
Unger [28] (2010)	72	–	–	63% at 1 year
Oshiro [29] (2010)	80	–	–	60% at 2 years
Baba [35] (2010)	90	72% at 3 years	82% at 3 years	66% at 3 years
Bradley [32] (2010)	86	75% at 2 years[a,b]	90% at 2 years[a,b]	86% at 2 years
Andratschke [34] (2011)	60	29% at 3 years	–	64% at 3 years
Haasbeek [32] (2011)	105	64% at 3 years	–	93% at 3 years
Bral [23] (2011)	150	–	–	Crude rate 94%
Olsen [38] (2011)	100	–	–	100% at 2 years [c]
Rowe [37] (2012)	114	–	–	94% at 2 years
Nuyttens [30] (2012)	132	53% at 3 years[b]	3 years 80%	76% at 2 years
Janssen [31] (2012)	77	–	–	87% at 1 year[a]

Biologically equivalent tumour dose (BED_{10}). Survival outcomes for central early-stage NSCLC. Local control for all central lung tumours receiving SABR

[a] Includes central and peripheral tumours with multivariate analysis showing location had no impact on outcome.

[b] Outcome not reported specifically but estimated from Kaplan–Meier curve.

[c] Local control at 2-years using 45 and 50 Gy in five fractions was 50% and 100%, respectively ($p = 0.006$).

Thirty month results of this study show no significant differences in regional recurrence (RR), locoregional recurrence (LRR), distant metastasis or freedom from any failure between the two groups. SBRT reduced the risk of local recurrence (LR) 4% versus 20 % for wedge but the difference is not significant (p=.07). Overall survival is better with wedge resection (87% wedge vs. 72% SBRT; p=0.01) but cause-specific survival (CSS), eliminating non cancer deaths, was identical (94% wedge vs. 93% SBRT; p= .53). The difference in overall survival is probably explained because patients undergoing SBRT were older with a higher comorbidity score.

SBRT Compare to Radiofrequency

Another therapeutic option for the treatment of Stage I-II NSCLC or pulmonary metastases is the Radiofrequency Ablation (RFA). Lung RFA need the establishment of a radiofrequency antenna in contact with the lesion to be treated, usually by transthoracic tomodensitometry guided puncture under general anesthesia. Local control described in the literature appears similar SBRT for peripheral lesions, but there is no comparative study available. For a larger analysis of results of RFA vs. SBRT, please refer to the paragraph "other local treatment".

Other Lung Indication

CyberKnife, due to its tracking capabilities, can be proposed for patients with a very low pulmonary capacity, even after pneumonectomy.

Stage III Tumors

Patients with stage IIIA or IIIB lung cancer may benefit from high doses of irradiation, and we know that chemoradiotherapy can cause inoperable tumors to become operable and increase overall patient survival. For these patients, NSCLC could be sterilized when conventional techniques and fractionation schemes.

For patients who responding to chemoradiotherapy and those who have locoregional well defined disease, an increase of dose can be proposed, with a boost by Cyberknife.

Reirradiation

For patients presenting non operable localized NSCLC, conventional radiotherapy or radiochemotherapy is often used. In cases of local relapse within or in the vicinity of the original radiation field, it is possible to do a reirradiation. But, in most of the cases, and to avoid toxicity to organ at risk, SBRT is used. This technique can be proposed in cases of NSCLC and SCLC

Lung Metastasis

There are no randomized trials evaluating the benefit of resection in patients with pulmonary metastases. However, multiple case reports and small series suggest that resection prolongs survival for oligometastatic patients. Slow growing bronchopulmonary metastases ($\leq$ 3 per lung) with controlled primary tumors are an indication of CyberKnife. Radiation patterns are generally the same as those of the primary tumors. There is discussion about the interest and the size of margin (see annex B). Preliminary results show a good local control, low toxicity and good quality of life.

Autopsy series have analyzed the frequency of lung metastases. These are present in 20-54% of all patients who die of cancer. The incidence of lung metastases varies during the evolution of cancer. At the presentation, the incidence is lower than in the autopsy series and varies depending on the primary tumor (see Table 3). In order of frequency of occurrence, we find breast cancer, colon, prostate, pancreas, kidney, thyroid, stomach, melanoma, ovarian, sarcomas.

Recently, Oh [19] have analyzed the treatment outcomes of SBRT, for patients with single or oligometastasis to the lungs. Sixty-seven metastatic lung lesions in 57 patients were treated with SBRT, the lungs were the most common primary organ, followed by the head and neck and the liver. Fractionation schedules were 50 Gy/5 fractions, 60 Gy/5 fractions and 60 Gy/4 fractions. Local tumor progression was 4.5%. The three-year actuarial local control rate was 94.5%. Tumors larger than or equal to 2.5 cm showed poorer local control. Metastatic tumors from the liver and colorectum showed lower local control rates than those from other organs. The two-year overall survival rate was 57.2%. Patients with disease-free intervals longer than two years showed a trend toward good prognosis (71.1% vs. 51.1% at two-year, p

=0.106). Grade 2 lung toxicity occurred in four patients (6.0%). One patient experienced Grade 5 lung toxicity.

Table 3. Frequency of primitive tumor in autopsy series

Primary Tumor	Frequency at Presentation, %	Frequency at Autopsy, %
Choriocarcinoma	60	70-100
Melanoma	5	66-80
Testis, germ cell	12	70-80
Osteosarcoma	15	75
Thyroid	7	65
Kidney	20	50-75
Head and neck	5	15-40
Breast	4	60
Bronchus	30	40
Colorectal	< 5	25-40
Prostate	5	15-50
Bladder	7	25-30
Uterus	< 1	30-40
Cervix	< 5	20-30
Pancreas	< 1	25-40
Esophagus	< 1	20-35
Stomach	< 1	20-35
Ovary	5	oct-25
Hepatoma	< 1	20-60

SBRT for single or oligo-metastasis to the lung seems quite effective and safe. Tumor size, disease-free interval, and presence of extrathoracic disease are prognosticators for survival.

When metastasis is detected, the frequency of the involved organ is presented (without lungs) in table 4.

Table 4. Frequency of pathology for lung metastasis

Organ	Frequency (%)
Breast cancer	19
Oesophagus/stomach cancer and colon/rectum cancer	17
Kidney and bladder	10
Genital cancer	10
Osteosarcoma and sarcoma	9
Head and neck cancer	4
Thyroid cancer	3
Prostate cancer	2
Others	6
unknown origin	15

Other Indications

CK utilizes the Synchrony® Respiratory Tracking System that precisely identifies the tumor location during breathing; it can be used in case of:

- Up-front treatment of obstructing endobronchial lesion with c post-obstructive pneumonia
- Pain metastasis in one or more fractions in cases of reirradiation.
- Clinical research

Stage III (boost)
Stage II lesion (mediastinal 3DRT and SBRT on primitive tumor)

Conclusion

Presents indication of CK for the lung cancer can be summarized:

Primitive Tumors

Stage I medically inoperable
Patients stage I who refuse surgery

Stage III for a boost (research or after clinical case discussion)
Lung tumor reirradiation
Recurrence on unique lung

Secondary Tumor

Oligo metastatic patient with a slow growing profile

Others Treatment

Pain metastasis
Obstructing endobronchial lesion
Clinical research

References

[1] Mountain CF. The international system for staging lung cancer. *Semin Surg Oncol.* 2000 Mar;18(2):106-15.

[2] Naruke T, Tsuchiya R, Kondo H et al. Prognosis and survival after resection for bronchogenic carcinoma based on the 1997 TNM-staging classification: the Japanese experience. *Ann Thorac Surg.* 2001 Jun;71(6):1759-64.

[3] Uematsu M, Shioda A, Suda A et al. Computed tomography-guided frameless stereotactic radiotherapy for stage I non-small cell lung cancer: a 5-year experience. *Int J Radiat Oncol Biol Phys.* 2001 Nov 1;51(3):666-70.

[4] Nagata Y, Takayama K, Matsuo Y et al. Clinical outcomes of a phase I/II study of 48 Gy of stereotactic body radiotherapy in 4 fractions for primary lung cancer using a stereotactic body frame. *Int J Radiat Oncol Biol Phys.* 2005 Dec 1;63(5):1427-31. Epub 2005 Sep 19.

[5] Fukumoto S, Shirato H, Shimsu S et al. Small-volume image-guided radiotherapy using hypofractionated, coplanar, and noncoplanar multiple fields for patients with inoperable Stage I nonsmall cell lung carcinomas. *Cancer.* 2002 Oct 1;95(7):1546-53.

[6] Onishi H, Kuriyama K, Komiyama T et al. Clinical outcomes of stereotactic radiotherapy for stage I non-small cell lung cancer using a

novel irradiation technique: patient self-controlled breath-hold and beam switching using a combination of linear accelerator and CT scanner. *Lung Cancer*. 2004 Jul;45(1):45-55.

[7] Hof H, Herfarth KK, Münter M, Hoess A et al. Stereotactic single-dose radiotherapy of stage I non-small-cell lung cancer (NSCLC). *Int J Radiat Oncol Biol Phys*. 2003 Jun 1;56(2):335-41.

[8] McGarry RC, Papiez L, Williams M et al. Stereotactic body radiation therapy of early-stage non-small-cell lung carcinoma: phase I study. *Int J Radiat Oncol Biol Phys*. 2005 Nov 15;63(4):1010-5. Epub 2005 Aug 22.

[9] Wulf J, Haedinger U, Oppitz U et al. Stereotactic radiotherapy for primary lung cancer and pulmonary metastases: a noninvasive treatment approach in medically inoperable patients. *Int J Radiat Oncol Biol Phys*. 2004 Sep 1;60(1):186-96.

[10] Onishi H, Shirato H, Nagata Y et al. Hypofractionated stereotactic radiotherapy (HypoFXSRT) for stage I non-small cell lung cancer: updated results of 257 patients in a Japanese multi-institutional study. *J Thorac Oncol*. 2007 Jul;2(7 Suppl 3):S94-100.

[11] Onishi H, Shirato H, Nagata Y et al. Stereotactic body radiotherapy (SBRT) for operable stage I non-small-cell lung cancer: can SBRT be comparable to surgery? *Int J Radiat Oncol Biol Phys*. 2011 Dec 1;81(5):1352-8. doi: 10.1016/j.ijrobp.2009.07.1751. Epub 2010 Jul 16.

[12] Fakiris AJ, McGarry RC, Yiannoutsos et al. Stereotactic body radiation therapy for early-stage non-small-cell lung carcinoma: four-year results of a prospective phase II study. *Int J Radiat Oncol Biol Phys*. 2009 Nov 1;75(3):677-82

[13] Timmerman R, Paulus R, Galvin J et al. Stereotactic body radiation therapy for inoperable early stage lung cancer. *JAMA*. 2010 Mar 17;303(11):1070-6.

[14] Haasbeek CJ, Lagerwaard FJ, Slotman BJ et al. Outcomes of stereotactic ablative radiotherapy for centrally located early-stage lung cancer. *J Thorac Oncol*. 2011 Dec;6(12):2036-43.

[15] Van der Voort van Zyp NC, Prévost JB, Hoogeman MS et al. Stereotactic radiotherapy with real-time tumor tracking for non-small cell lung cancer: clinical outcome. *Radiother Oncol*. 2009 Jun;91(3):296-300.

[16] Senthi S, Haasbeek C.J.A, Slotman B.J et al. Outcomes of stereotatic ablative radiotherapy for central tumours : a systematic review In press *Radiother oncol* (2013), http://dx.doi.org/10.1016/j.radonc.2013.01.004

[17] Grills IS, Mangona VS, Welsh R et al. Outcomes after stereotactic lung radiotherapy or wedge resection for stage I non-small-cell lung cancer. *J Clin Oncol.* 2010 Feb 20;28(6):928-35.

[18] Sher DJ, Wee JO, Punglia RS. Cost-effectiveness analysis of stereotactic body radiotherapy and radiofrequency ablation for medically inoperable, early-stage non-small cell lung cancer. *Int J Radiat Oncol Biol Phys.* 2011 Dec 1;81(5):e767-74.

[19] Oh D, Ahn YC, Seo JM, Shin EH, Park HC, Lim do H, Pyo H.Potentially curative stereotactic body radiation therapy (SBRT) for single or oligometastasis to the lung. *Acta Oncol.* 2012 May;51(5):596-602.

Part IIa: Technique

In: The Revolution of Robotic ...
Editor: Pierre-Yves Bondiau
ISBN: 978-1-62808-718-5

Chapter 5

Radiobiology and Its Applications to Stereotactic Body Radiotherapy

Adel Courdi[1,2,*]
[1]Department of Radiation Oncology, Antoine-Lacassagne Cancer Center, Nice, France
[2]University of Nice Sophia-Antipolis, Nice, France

Abstract

Ionizing radiation produces DNA damage, mostly single and double-strand breaks, leading to cell death, or sometimes mutation, in the absence of correct repair. With conventional radiotherapy, because normal tissues are equally hit as tumor cells, dose fractionation allows greater repair of radiation damage by normal cells than by tumor cells. Radiotherapy with curative intent delivers low doses per fraction in multiple fractions to spare normal tissues in the field. The end-effect depends on many factors such as intrinsic radiosensitivity, amount of repair, tumor hypoxia, cell proliferation kinetics and the irradiated volume. Depending on whether normal tissues are arranged serially or in parallel, the damage will be sensitive to maximal dose or dose-volume histogram, respectively. Because stereotactic body radiotherapy (SBRT)

* E-mail: adel.courdi@nice.unicancer.fr.

is a highly precise technique greatly sparing normal tissues, high doses per fraction given in a very few fractions (hypofractionation) can be safely given. Concerning normal tissues, the linear quadratic (LQ) model is generally applied to derive equivalences to standard fractionation, for estimating late effects. However, tumor cells receive doses that fall beyond the limits of application of the LQ model, ant its use may lead to inaccurate estimation of the amount of cell kill. New mechanisms of action at very high doses are currently investigated.

The dose distribution of SBRT is not likely to modify the current knowledge about second radiation-induced cancer. Progress in radiobiology and extended patient follow-up will help refining estimates of the benefits and hazards of SBRT.

Introduction

The basic mechanisms of radiation-induced damage are essentially the same whether normal tissues or tumors are involved. Because water molecules are the main constituents of the mammalian body, radiation effects are mostly the consequences of the ionization of H_2O as an initial event. Initial water ionization is particularly the case for the high-energy X-rays that are produced by accelerators (such as those used for stereotactic body radiotherapy). This process is called an "indirect effect," as opposed to a "direct effect," which is observed with particles with high ionization densities that have the power to ionize biological molecules as a primary event.

Although many chemical reactions are encountered when water molecules are ionized, the formation of the hydroxyl radical "$OH^{\cdot}$" is an important step in producing a biological effect. $OH^{\cdot}$ carries a high oxidation capacity due to its removal of hydrogen from biological compounds. This type of damage can be chemically repaired if hydrogen-giving molecules are available in the environment. In contrast, the presence of oxygen will help fixate radiation damage and is thus considered the most important radiation sensitizer. Alternatively, the lack of oxygen tends to reduce the magnitude of radiation effects and contributes to radiation resistance and protection.

Radiation damage affects all constituents of the cell, but the main target of significance is the nuclear DNA. Damage to the nuclear DNA can result in several kinds of lesions, such as base deletion, base replacement, base binding, or binding between base and proteins.

DNA breaks may be either single-strand or double-strand breaks. For example, a dose of one Gy leads to approximately 1000 single-strand breaks and 40 double-strand breaks. Despite this apparently large amount of damage, a cell hit by 1 Gy of X-rays is more likely to survive than to die. In fact, the powerful repair mechanisms that continuously prevail or only act during DNA replication can greatly wipe out radiation damage. However, faulty repair may also occur, resulting in different consequences. Disrepair can go unnoticed or be incompatible with cell survival (leading to the cell's death). A third possibility is that an erroneous repair can occur that does not induce cell death, but instead leads to cell transformation. And cell transformation may be the first step toward radiation carcinogenesis.

Structural changes are observed in chromosomes, namely in intra-chromosomal exchanges, inter-chromosomal translocations, terminal deletions, and ring formation among other lesions. The measurements of some of these aberrations can help estimate the whole body dose that a patient accidentally received.

Cell Death after Irradiation

Two main modes of cell death are observed after its exposure to ionizing radiation. First, its death by apoptosis may be observed in as few as 6 hours after irradiation. Its demise is activated by a death signal and influenced by a number of enzymes. It is a sort of programmed cell death that is useful in eliminating abnormal cells. More often, however, a cell dies after one of its successive mitoses. This mitotic or delayed cell death has been widely studied by measuring the capacity of a cell to form viable daughter cells for an extended period of long time. Survival curves are the graphic expression of the relationship between the fraction of surviving cells and the radiation dose. The model that best fits the experimental points is the linear-quadratic (LQ) model (where S is the surviving fraction and d is the dose per fraction):

$$S = e^{-(\alpha d+\beta d^2)} \qquad (1)$$

This model implies that cell mortality may be the result of single-track events ($e^{-\alpha d}$) or two-track events ($e^{-\beta d^2}$). Single-track mortality prevails at low doses and low dose rates. The dose at which the single-track mortality (the linear term) equals the double-track mortality (the quadratic term) equals α/β. The α/β ratio is widely used to establish biological equivalences between different fractionation schemes and reflects the bending of the survival curve. If the ratio is high, it indicates that the linear term predominates at clinically relevant doses; in other words, cell mortality is more or less proportional to dose. A low α/β ratio, however, signifies continuous bending of the curve, with a higher-than-linear effect at high doses [1].

If considering the effect as equaling –Log(S), equation (1) becomes:

$$E = \alpha d + \beta d^2 \tag{2}$$

Figure 1 displays the dose-effect relationship for early-reacting tissues, late-reacting tissues, and several tumors. The low α/β ratio of late-reacting tissues is responsible for the sharp bending of the curve. The significance of that bending is that late-responding tissues are highly sensitive to modifications of the dose per fraction. If a fractionation scheme must be modified, it is thus very useful to know the α/β ratio of a particular tissue and tumor [2].

Biological Factors Influencing Radiation Response

The end result of radiotherapy on a tumor population depends on several factors:

The Intrinsic Radiation Resistance of Tumor Cells

Independent of other environmental factors, tumor cells respond differently to ionizing radiation. It has long been demonstrated that their response depends on the histological tumor type (whether irradiation is carried out in vivo or in vitro) [3, 4]. Embryonal tumors are among the most sensitive and melanomas and gliomas are among the most resistant; lung tumors are moderately sensitive. Within lung tumors, small cell carcinomas are more sensitive than other tumor cell types. Studies are in progress to determine the genetic causes of why different cells have different responses to radiation.

Repair of Radiation Damage

Conventional radiotherapy is conducted with fractionated doses. Dose fractionation allows for the repair of radiation damage between fractions, a process which is considered to be more efficient in normal tissues than in tumor cells.

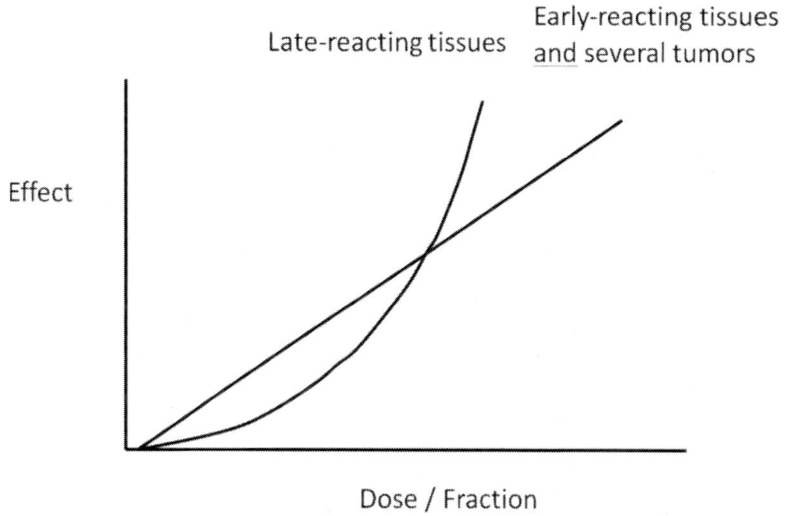

Figure 1. Schematic dose-effect relationship in normal tissues and tumors.

A time interval of 6-8 hours between fractions allows for the complete recovery of radiation damage. Late-reactive tissues, however, have a slow-repair component and could be further damaged by small time intervals between fractions.

Tumor Hypoxia

It has been demonstrated that animal and human tumors may contain hypoxic cells. Vascular constriction may lead to acute hypoxia, and increasing the distance between tumor cells and blood vessels contributes to chronic hypoxia. Tumor hypoxia makes the tumor less responsive. Fractionation, however, favors the re-oxygenation of tumors and thus reduces their radioresistance. Particle radiation with high ionization densities are less dependent on oxygen and are used advantageously in hypoxic tumors.

Tumor Proliferation

Cell proliferation kinetics are an important determinant in tumor radiotherapy. Although highly proliferating tumor cells respond more to radiation in the short term than do slowly proliferating cells [5], their high proliferation negatively affects the prognosis [6]. A positive correlation has been demonstrated between doubling times of pulmonary metastases and patient survival [7]. Moreover, because conventional radiotherapy schemes extend over several weeks, this extension offers tumor cells the time to oppose cell mortality and depletion by accelerating their repopulation. During the last weeks of radiotherapy, the effective dose per fraction is thus diminished as a substantial amount of its effectiveness is lost to counterbalancing tumor repopulation. Fractionation schemes that reduce the overall time of radiation are designed to offset the influence of accelerated tumor repopulation.

The Volume Effect

The results of radiotherapy are influenced by both the tumor volume and the volume of normal tissues that is being irradiated [8-11]. The higher the tumor volume, the higher the number of clonogens in the tumor, and the lower the tumor control probability (TCP). Additionally, the volume of the irradiated normal tissues is a limiting factor. Damage to normal tissues can be estimated using normal tissue complication probability (NTCP) models as a function of the absorbed dose in a partial organ volume [12]. Normal tissues are organized in serial or parallel functional subunits (FSU). When these independent structures are damaged, the resulting organ failure will depend on whether these FSUs are arranged in series or in parallel [13].

Table 1 compares the characteristics that differentiate how different organs respond to radiation. An organ organized in parallel FSUs, such as the lung, will sustain severe damage in a small volume, but undergo moderate damage in a large volume. In contrast, a serially organized organ, such as the spinal cord, will be damaged by a high dose to a small volume, but be spared after exposure to a moderate dose, even to a large volume.

Table 1. Organization of FSUs in tissues

Organization	Serial	Parallel
Example	Spinal cord	Lung
Inducing damage	High dose even in a small volume	Moderate dose in a large volume
Relevant item	D_{max}	Dose volume histogram (DVH)

Hypofractionation and Stereotactic Body Radiation Therapy

Hypofractionation refers to when the total dose is delivered in fewer fractions than the 25-35 daily fractions of 2 Gy that is used by standard fractionation. The use of fewer fractions usually decreases the overall time of a patient's exposure to radiation. However, hypofractionation uses a higher dose per fraction (d/f) in order to compensate for the reduced total dose. Because late-reacting tissues are more easily damaged with a high d/f, they constitute a limiting factor to this scheme. Moreover, because normal tissues and tumors do not have the same dose-effect relationship (Figure 1), any change in the d/f will need different adjustments to the total dose. Figure 2 presents iso-effect lines between total dose and d/f. In this schematic representation, increasing the d/f necessitates reducing the total dose in order to keep the effect constant. Parallel curves indicate different endpoints. The dark lines, which represent early effects and many tumors, have shallower slopes than the red lines, which signify late-reacting tissues. A steep slope indicates that if the d/f is increased, the total dose should be greatly reduced in order to keep late effects constant. In that case, however, the tumor would be underdosed.

This graph shows how much the total dose needs to be reduced when the d/f is increased. If the d/f is changed from 2 Gy to 4 Gy, a moderate decrease in the total dose would be required for similar tumor control or a similar early effect (dark lines). A similar late effect (red lines) would necessitate a sharper decrease in the total dose. Nonetheless, hypofractionation plays an increasing role in modern radiotherapy.

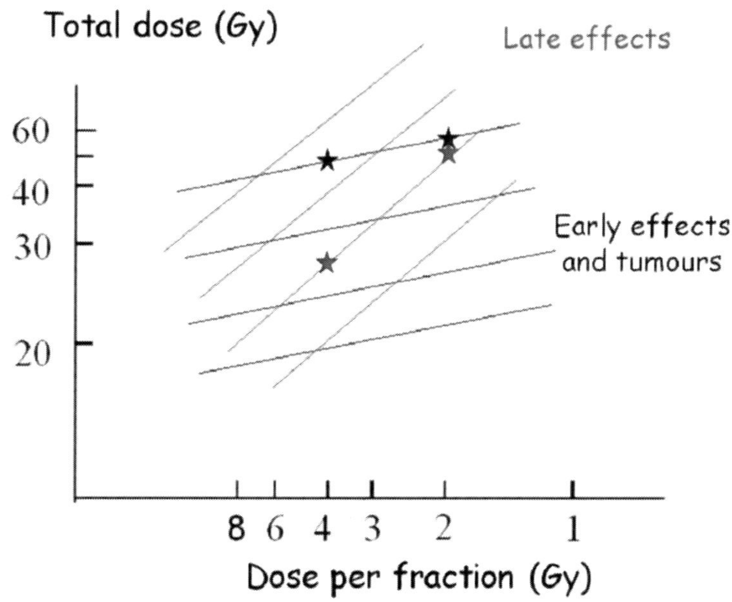

Figure 2. Iso-effect lines between total dose and dose per fraction.

Indications for Hypofractionation

Conventional Radiotherapy Techniques

With conventional radiotherapy techniques, normal tissues around the tumor receive almost the same dose as the tumor.

1. In cases where normal tissue tolerance dose is not reached and/or tumor cure is not the aim. This is particularly the case for palliative radiotherapy (e.g., a bone metastasis that would receive 8 Gy in one fraction or 13 Gy in 2 fractions).
2. Small treatment volume. A typical example is found when a small skin cancer is treated with electron beams or low-energy X-rays. Few normal tissue cells are present in the irradiated volume. Moreover, epithelial tissues have a high migratory capacity that contributes to the rapid healing of the normal skin tissues.

Structures that are arranged in a parallel type, such as the lung, are very sensitive to the volume effect. Lung tolerance doses are given in Table 2 [14].

Table 2. Dosimetric values associated with a 10% risk of radiation pneumonitis

Variable	Value
Mean lung dose	< 13 Gy < 10 Gy upper tumor 2 Gy lower tumor
V20 *	< 30% of lung volume
V30 **	< 20% of lung volume

* V20 refers to the lung volume that will receive ≥ 20 Gy. ** V30 refers to the lung volume that will receive ≥ 30 Gy.

3. Cases where the tumor has a low α/β ratio. Because high α/β ratios of about 10 Gy are found in epithelial head and neck tumors [15], these tumors are thus relatively insensitive to changes in fractionation (e.g., hypofractionation).

However, the normal tissues that surround these tumors have low α/β ratios, and hypofractionation will lead to late normal tissue damage at constant tumor control. Because of this damage, hypofractionation does not bring any advantage when it is used to treat head and neck tumors. Not all tumors, however, present high α/β ratios. For instance, breast [16], prostate [17], and probably melanoma [18] and sarcomas [19] have low α/β ratios.

If the α/β ratio of the tumor is lower than that of the late-reacting normal tissues, hypofractionation will benefit the patient, offering fewer late reactions at equal tumor control.

Unconventional Radiotherapy Techniques

The phrase "Unconventional radiotherapy techniques" refers to special techniques that can be adopted when the normal tissues around the tumor receive a lower dose than the tumor itself.

1. High dose rate brachytherapy. The implantation of sealed radioactive sources within the tumor volume allows for a high dose to be

delivered to that volume (Figure 3). The dose gradient falls rapidly outside that volume, sparing normal tissues. Hypofractionation can therefore be done safely.

2. Charged-particle radiotherapy. The physical characteristics of charged particles as protons or carbon ions differ from X-rays or gamma-rays. Maximum ionization, and therefore dose delivery, occurs at a certain depth (Bragg peak) before stopping of the particles.
   Normal tissues situated before the Bragg peak receive a lower dose, and those situated after the peak are completely spared. Therefore, the volume of normal tissues that will receive a significant dose is greatly reduced (Figure 4).
   Patients treated with particle beams receive hypofractionated radiation therapy.

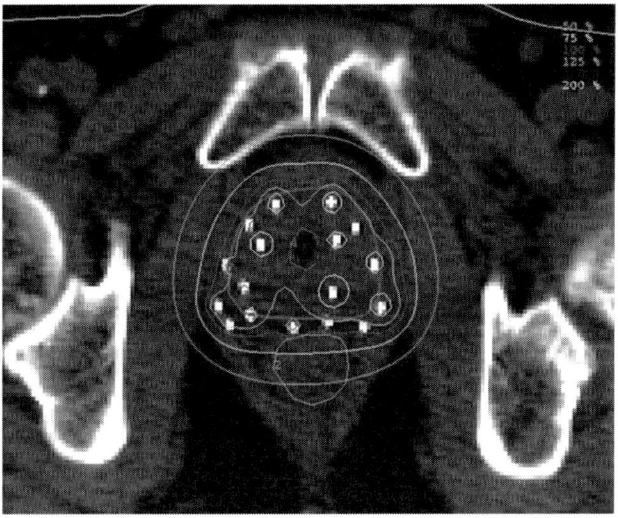

Figure 3. High-dose rate brachytherapy in prostate cancer.

Advantages of Hypofractionation

1) Possibility of increasing the tumor dose; 2) reducing overall treatment time; 3) improving patient comfort; 4) reducing travel; 5) allowing more patients to be treated

Dose equivalences with SBRT

3 – Stereotactic radiotherapy. Advances in radiotherapy techniques have made possible the sharp conformation of the isodoses to the treatment volume. The volume of normal tissues that receive significant doses has been greatly reduced due to, among other options, the use of multiple sources and/or angles of treatment, and the elaboration of dose constraints to normal tissues (Figure 5). Because there is no longer any danger that normal tissues will receive high doses per fraction, there is no obstacle to the use of hypofractionation. With respect to hypofractionation's effects on lung toxicity, today's highly conformal dose distributions are radiobiologically more forgiving [20, 21]. It has also been reported that the overall survival of patients with pulmonary metastatic nodules was improved using hypofractionated SBRT with high biologically equivalent dose (BED) values [22].

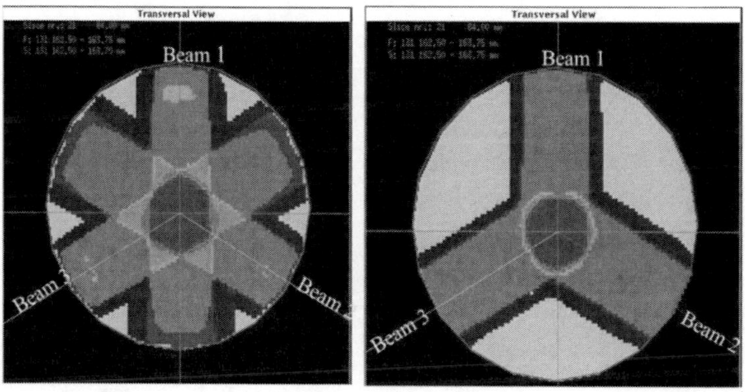

Figure 4. The dosimetry OF 3 beams of high-energy. X-Rays (left) compared to 3 beams of high-energy protons (right).

Normal Tissues Equivalence

Because SBRT uses high doses per fraction, it is highly desirable to convert SBRT's total dose to the equivalent dose that would be given in a classic 2 Gy per fraction schedule. The LQ model can help in such conversion (at least in the case of late-reacting normal tissues, which are the limiting factor in radiotherapy practice).

If n fractions are given, the equation (2) (given before) can be written:

$$E = n(\alpha d + \beta d^2) = \alpha D + \beta dD \quad (3)$$

where D is the total dose.

The BED is defined as:

$$BED = E/\alpha = D\,(1 + d/(\alpha/\beta)) \quad (4)$$

A BED contains the dose unit and is considered to be the dose that would be given in an infinite number of fractions that yield the same effect. In other words, 2 different fractionation schemes that have the same BED will have the same effect. For late effects the time factor is negligible, and the formula can be applied to fractionation schemes that have different overall durations.

To calculate a total BED, add a BED value that was derived from a certain fractionation (e.g., conventional fractionation) to a BED value that was derived from a different scheme (e.g., SBRT).

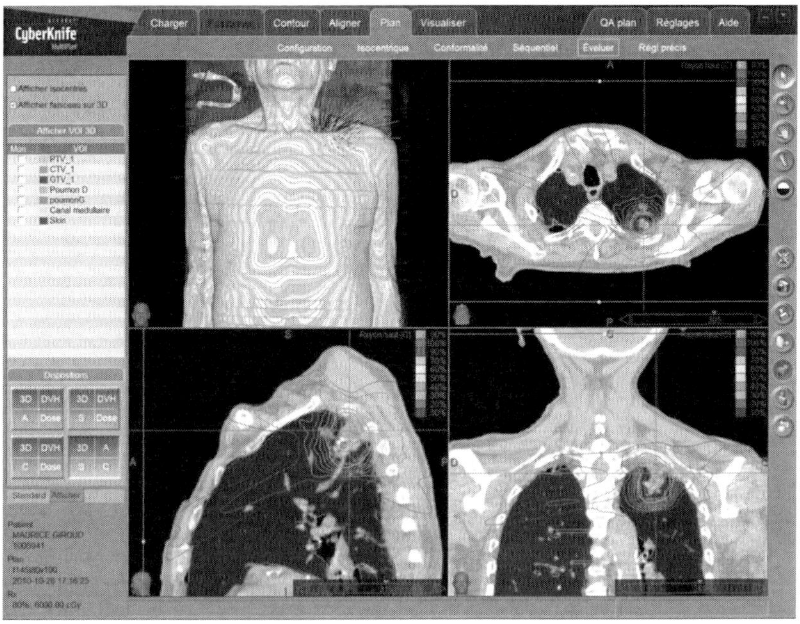

Figure 5. An upper lobe lung tumor treated with stereotactic radiotherapy.

To calculate BED, the α/β ratio has to be known. For most late effects, an α/β ratio of 3 Gy is appropriate. The spinal cord has an α/β ratio close to 2 Gy.

The following schemes have the same BED and, therefore, have the same effect on late-reacting tissues with an α/β ratio of 3 Gy: 18 fractions of 2 Gy, 10 fractions of 3 Gy, and 2 fractions of 8 Gy.

The LQ model is inappropriate for high doses per fraction. Above 10 Gy, the model would be expected to become progressively less accurate [23]. Also, it does not take into account the critical molecular, cellular, and tissue effects that are produced at high doses per fraction [24]. Despite these limitations, this model may be applied to normal tissues that were exposed to SBRT because the doses per fraction received by these tissues are within the limits for use of the LQ model.

When comparing a fractionation scheme to one using standard fractionation, it is more practical to use the total dose that is equivalent to 2 Gy per fraction (or EQD_2) than the BED. If the 2 schedules are equivalent, and according to equation (2) (where d and D stand for d_2 and D_2 in the unconventional fractionation:

$$\alpha D_1 + \beta d_1 D_1 = \alpha D_2 + \beta d_2 D_2 \quad (5)$$

Setting EQD_2 as D_1 and $d_1 = 2$:

$$EQD_2 = D \,.\, (d + (\alpha/\beta)) \,/\, (2 + (\alpha/\beta)) \quad \textbf{(6)}$$

Tumor Equivalence

Whereas the values of α/β ratios for most late-reacting tissues are known with good confidence, only a few α/β ratios have been reported for tumors. Head and neck tumors, for example, have been determined to have high α/β ratios of close to 10 Gy. Epithelial tumors also probably share a high α/β ratio. Likewise, because adenocarcinomas such as breast [16] and prostate [17] tumors have low α/β ratios, other adenocarcinomas probably behave similarly. It is therefore hypothesized that lung tumors will have high or low α/β ratios according to whether their pathological type is epithelial or adenocarcinoma, respectively.

A further point to consider is that tumors in the lung may be secondary. In that case, metastatic tumors of the lung will share the α/β ratio of the primary tumor, and equivalences will differ accordingly.

When planning tumor radiotherapy, it is important to factor in the additional variable of time. It was established many years ago that the total duration of fractionated radiotherapy, especially for head and neck tumors, needs to be considered into account. Specifically, the extension of overall treatment time due to substantial interruptions is an adverse prognostic factor. In other words, tumor cells accelerate their repopulation if several weeks pass between the first and the last sessions [25].

To include the time factor in the LQ model, one needs to know the value of α, and the potential doubling time (T_{pot}) of the tumor; Equation (2) becomes (where T is the overall treatment time):

$$E = \alpha D + \beta dD - Ln\ 2\ .\ T\ /\ T_{pot} \tag{7}$$

and equation (4) for BED becomes:

$$E/\alpha = BED = D\ (1 + d/(\alpha/\beta)) - Ln\ 2\ .\ T\ /\ (\alpha T_{pot})$$

T_{pot} has been calculated for some tumors and could be as short as a few days or vary widely. Furthermore, it has been demonstrated that tumor cell repopulation is triggered at 3 or 4 weeks after the start of irradiation and some investigators use $T - T_k$ instead of T where T_k is the triggering repopulation time [25]. Parameter α is not precisely known, but depends on the intrinsic sensitivity of the tumor.

Due to the above-mentioned considerations, a simple way to include the time factor in the LQ model is to first calculate the EQD_2 and to then apply a modification factor which takes into account the difference in overall treatment times between the 2 schedules and the amount of dose lost per day due to cell proliferation ($D_{prolif.}$).

$$EQD_{2,T} = EQD_{2t} - (T - t)\ D_{prolif.} \tag{8}$$

D_{prolif} is around 0.6 Gy/day in head and neck epithelial tumors, and probably less in other tumors. Because SBRT is delivered in a short overall time, the time factor should be taken into consideration for if tumor equivalences are compared with long overall time schedules.

Applied to SBRT, the uncertainties of these equivalences are illustrated in Table 3.

As previously mentioned, the LQ model is not reliable when applied to high doses per fraction, and the equivalences in Table 3, especially when used with a dose per fraction as high as 20 Gy, may thus be incorrect.

Table 3. EQD_2 variations according to α/β and the time factor

SBRT dose	EQD_2			
	Squamous cell carcinoma $\alpha/\beta = 10$	With time factor $\alpha/\beta = 10$	Adenocarcinoma $\alpha/\beta = 4$	Sarcoma $\alpha/\beta = 2$
3 x 20 = 60 Gy	150	191	240	330
5 x 15 = 75 Gy	156	198	237	319

Table 4. Terminal slopes after high doses to a variety of tissues

Tissue	D_0 (Gy)	Reference
Cartilage growth plate	1.65	[26, 27]
Skin	1.3 – 1.4	[28]
Colon	1.42	[29]
Spermatogenic tubules	1.74	[30]
Telogen hair follicles	1.35	[31]
Kidney tubules	1.25	[32]

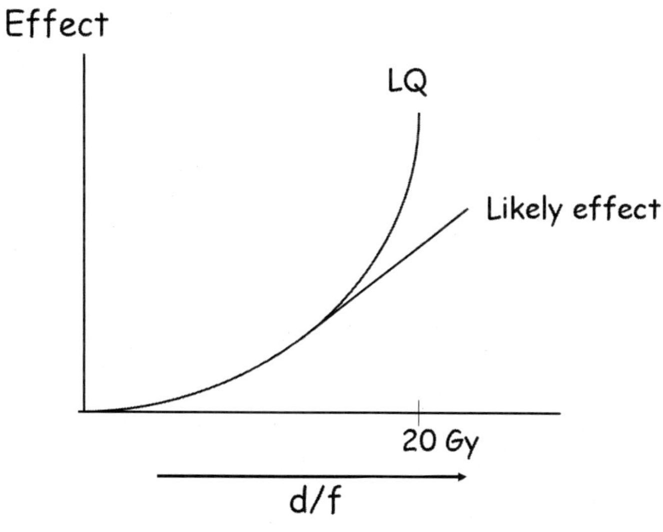

Figure 6. The effect at high doses per fraction may not be quadratic.

Some experiments have demonstrated that survival curves from in vivo assays are linear at high doses. The terminal linear segment is characterized by D_0, which is inversely related to the slope of the curve (Table 4).

The practical implication of a terminal slope is that the LQ may overestimate the effect at high doses per fraction (Figure 6).

Other models that intend to approximate the effects observed at high doses are being evaluated. These models include the universal survival-curve [33], two-component (TC) [34], generalized LQ [35], and linear-quadratic-cubic (LQC) [36].

Although these models can hardly describe the complex biological processes that cell undergo after radiation, they can help design optimal treatment plans.

In addition, at high doses, other factors should be considered: no expression of re-oxygenation, activation of vascular endothelial damage, obliteration of abnormal vasculature, and the possible occurrence of CD8 + T-cell dependent effects.

Ultimately, however, ideal dose and fractionation will be based on clinical experiences and prospective trials that consider both tumor efficacy and normal tissue toxicity.

SBRT and Radiation Carcinogenesis

Much information has accumulated pertaining to the effects of radiation carcinogenesis following standard radiotherapy [37, 38]. These data suggest that a patient's susceptibility to secondary cancer particularly depends upon the following characteristics: age at exposure, genetics, how much volume was irradiated, the dose given to that irradiated volume, associated treatments, and tissue susceptibility. Because radiation-induced cancer arises after a long latency period that may extend for the whole patient's life, no data are available that pertain to modern radiotherapy techniques [39].

Using a mathematical model that considered cell kill and mutation, a study has suggested that hypofractionation may better reduce second cancer occurrence than standard fractionation [40].

Another recent study has estimated cancer risk per unit mass of irradiated normal tissue based on integral dose calculation and the observed secondary cancer incidence in a cohort of 5000 survivors of childhood cancer [41]. It has been shown that the risk increases with the dose and the irradiated mass (volume). Compared to conventional radiotherapy, the volume receiving a dose higher than 40 Gy (high risk per unit dose) is smaller with SBRT, and the volume receiving a dose lower than 5 Gy (low risk per unit dose) is larger. Therefore, the risks are balanced on each side. In addition, it is worth noting that the volume receiving an ablative dose cannot develop secondary cancer, due to total cell kill. Taken together, it is unlikely that SBRT will lead to more secondary cancers than conventional radiotherapy.

References

[1] Courdi A. Le modèle linéaire-quadratique et ses applications à la radiothérapie. *J. Chim. Phys.* 1994; 91:1025-40.

[2] Bentzen SM, Joiner MC. The linear-quadratic approach in clinical practice. In: Joiner and van der Kogel: *Basic Clinical Radiobiology*, 4th Edition, Hodder Arnold 2009; 120-34.

[3] Fertil, B, Malaise. Intrinsic radiosensitivity of human cell lines is correlated with radioresponsiveness of human tumors: analysis of 101 published survival curves. *Int. J. Radiat. Oncol. Biol. Phys.* 1985; 11: 1699-707.

[4] Fertil B, Dertinger H, Courdi A, Malaise EP. Mean inactivation dose: a useful concept for intercomparison of human survival curves. *Radiat. Res.* 1984; 99:73-84.

[5] Malaise EP, Chavaudra N, Guichard M, Courdi A, Vazquez T. The influence of tumor growth kinetics on the response of radiation therapy and drug therapy in man. In: *Antibiotics and Chemotherapy, Fundamentals in Cancer Chemotherapy,* vol. 23, Karger, Basel, 1978; 181-190.

[6] Tubiana M, Courdi A. Cell proliferation kinetics in human solid tumors: relation to probability of metastatic dissemination and long-term survival. *Radiother. Oncol.* 1989; 15:1-18.

[7] Malaise EP, Chavaudra N, Courdi A, Vazquez T. Tumor growth rate and pulmonary metastasis. In: Weiss & Gilbert: *Pulmonary Metastasis*; G. Hall & Co. Boston 1978; 200-220.

[8] Xue J, Goldman HW, Grimm J, et al. Dose-volume effects on brainstem dose tolerance in radiosurgery. *J. Neurosurg.* 2012; 117 Suppl:189-96.

[9] Mayo C, Martel MK, Marks LB, Flickinger J, Nam J, Kirkpatrick J. Radiation dose-volume effects of optic nerves and chiasm. *Int. J. Radiat. Oncol. Biol. Phys.* 2010; 76: S28-35.

[10] Vargas C, Martinez A, Kestin LL, et al. Dose-volume analysis of predictors for chronic rectal toxicity after treatment of prostate cancer with adaptive image-guided radiotherapy. *Int. J. Radiat. Oncol. Biol. Phys.* 2005; 62:1297-308.

[11] Werner-Wasik M, Yorke E, Deasy J, Nam J, Marks LB. Radiation dose-volume effects in the esophagus. *Int. J. Radiat. Oncol. Biol. Phys.* 2010; 76: S86-93.

[12] Lyman JT. Complication probability as assessed from dose-volume histograms. *Radiat. Res.* 1985; Suppl 8:S13-19.

[13] Withers HR, Taylor JM, Maciejewski B. Treatment volume and tissue tolerance. *Int. J. Radiat. Oncol. Biol. Phys.* 1988; 14:751-9.

[14] Ortholan C, Mornex F. Normal tissue tolerance to external beam radiation therapy: Lung. *Cancer/Radiother.* 2010; 14:312–18.

[15] Stuschke M, Thames HD. Fractionation sensitivities and dose-control relations of head and neck. *Radiother. Oncol.* 1999; 51:113-21.

[16] The START Trialists' Group. The UK Standardisation of Breast Radiotherapy (START) Trial A of radiotherapy hypofractionation for treatment of early breast cancer: a randomised trial. *Lancet Oncol* 2008; 9: 331–41.

[17] Brenner DJ, Martinez AA, Edmundson GK, Mitchell C, Thames HD, Armour EP. Direct evidence that prostate tumors show high sensitivity to fractionation (low alpha/beta ratio), similar to late-responding normal tissue. *Int. J. Radiat. Oncol. Biol. Phys.* 2002; 52:6-13.

[18] Bentzen SM, Overgaard J, Thames HD. Clinical radiobiology of malignant melanoma. *Radiother. Oncol.* 1989; 16:169-82.

[19] Thames HD, Suit HD. Tumor radioresponsiveness versus fractionation sensitivity. *Int. J. Radiat. Oncol. Biol. Phys.* 1986; 12:687-91.

[20] Vogelius IS, Westerly DC, Cannon GM, Bentzen SM. Hypofractionation does not increase radiation pneumonitis risk with modern conformal radiation delivery techniques. *Acta Oncol.* 2010; 49(7):1052-7.

[21] Jin JY, Kong FM, Chetty IJ, et al. Impact of fraction size on lung radiation toxicity: hypofractionation may be beneficial in dose escalation of radiotherapy for lung cancers. *Int. J. Radiat. Oncol. Biol. Phys.* 2010; 76:782-8.

[22] Casamassima F, Masi L, Bonucci I, et al. Relevance of biologically equivalent dose values in outcome evaluation of stereotactic radiotherapy for lung nodules. *Int. J. Radiat. Oncol. Biol. Phys.* 2008; 71: 145-51.

[23] Brenner DJ. The linear-quadratic model is an appropriate methodology for determining isoeffective doses at large doses per fraction. *Semin. Radiat. Oncol.* 2008; 18:234-9.

[24] Kirpatrick JP, Meyer JJ, Marks LB. The linear-quadratic model is inappropriate to model high dose per fraction effects in radiosurgery. *Semin. Radiat. Oncol.* 2008; 18:240-3.

[25] Withers HR, Taylor JM, Maciejewski B. The hazard of accelerated tumor clonogen repopulation during radiotherapy. *Acta Oncol.* 1988; 27: 131-46.

[26] Kember NF. An in vivo cell survival system based on the recovery of rat growth cartilage from radiation injury. *Nature.* 1965; 207:501-3.

[27] Kember NF. Cell survival and radiation damage in growth cartilage. *Br. J. Radiol.* 1967; 40: 496-505.

[28] Withers HR. The dose-survival relationship for irradiation of epithelial cells of mouse skin. *Br. J. Radiol.* 1967; 40:187-94.

[29] Withers HR, Mason K, Reid BO, et al. Response of mouse intestine to neutrons and gamma rays in relation to dose fractionation and division cycle. *Cancer.* 1974; 34:39-47.

[30] Withers HR, Hunter N, Barkley HT Jr, Reid BO. Radiation survival and regeneration characteristics of spermatogenic stem cells of mouse testis. *Radiat. Res.* 1974; 57:88-103.

[31] Griem ML, Dimitrievich GS, Lee RM. The effects of X-irradiation and adriamycin on proliferating and nonproliferating hair coat of the mouse. *Int. J. Radiat. Oncol. Biol. Phys.* 1979; 5:1261-4.

[32] Withers HR, Mason KA, Thames HD. Late radiation response of kidney assayed by tubule-cell survival. *Br. J. Radiol.* 1986; 59:587-95.

[33] Park C, Papiez L, Zhang S, Story M, Timmerman RD. Universal survival curve and single fraction equivalent dose: useful tools in understanding potency of ablative radiotherapy. *Int. J. Radiat. Oncol. Biol. Phys.* 2008; 70:847-52.

[34] Joiner M. The LQ model applicable for brachytherapy with large doses per fraction. *Radiother. Oncol.* 2008; Suppl 2:S9.

[35] Wang JZ, Huang Z, Lo SS, Yuh WT, Mayr NA. A generalized linear-quadratic model for radiosurgery, stereotactic body radiation therapy, and high-dose rate brachytherapy. *Sci. Transl. Med.* 2010; 2:39-48.

[36] Joiner MC. Quantifying cell kill and cell survival. In: Joiner and van der Kogel: *Basic Clinical Radiobiology*, 4th Edition, Hodder Arnold 2009; 41-55.

[37] Berrington de Gonzalez A, E Curtis RE, Kry SF, et al. Proportion of second cancers attributable to radiotherapy treatment in adults: a cohort study in the US SEER cancer registries. *Lancet Oncol.* 2011; 12:353-60.

[38] Doyen J, Courdi A, Gérard JP. Second primitive malignant neoplasm after radiotherapy. *Cancer Radiother*. 2010; 14: 255-62.

[39] Newhauser WD, Durante M. Assessing the risk of second malignancies after modern radiotherapy. *Nature Rev. Cancer* 2011; 11:438-448.

[40] Schneider U, Besserer J, Mack A. Hypofractionated radiotherapy has the potential for second cancer reduction. *Theor. Biol. Med. Model Biol.* 2010; 7:4.

[41] Tubiana M, Diallo I, Chavaudra J, et al. A new method of assessing the dose-carcinogenic effect relationship in patients exposed to ionizing radiation. A concise presentation of preliminary data. *Health Phys.* 2011; 100: 296-9.

In: The Revolution of Robotic ...
Editor: Pierre-Yves Bondiau
ISBN: 978-1-62808-718-5

Chapter 6

CyberKnife Description

Serge Marcié[1*], Karen Bénézery[1] and Pierre-Yves Bondiau[1,2]
[1]Department of Radiation Oncology, Antoine-Lacassagne Cancer Center, Nice, France
[2]University of Nice Sophia-Antipolis, Nice, France

Abstract

For nearly a century, radiotherapy has greatly benefited from the development of computer, imaging and therapeutic equipment. After using low energy X-rays, the arrival of linear accelerators equipped with multileaf collimators and portal imaging have led to therapeutic advances. Recent years have seen the advent of conformal radiotherapy with intensity modulation, to ensure better protection of organs at risk (OAR). But a revolution is under way with the arrival of robots that have gradually entered the medical world. They include the perception (medical images and information), action (precise positioning in space) and feedback. The robot is a programmable tool capable of performing specific actions, adapted and repeated in a given environment. These robots, originally from the industrial world, are gradually implemented on rigid or semi-rigid organs (bone, brain…) and gradually integrating the field of cardiology and abdominal surgery. CyberKnife is a robot with a linear accelerator for used for performing stereotactic radiotherapy. The

* Email: serge.marcie@nice.unicancer.fr.

first CyberKnife device was developed in the 1990s in the United States, in California, under the direction of John R. Adler at Stanford University Medical Center. The linear accelerator miniaturized is fixed to a robot's arm, which has a high re-positioning accuracy, with six degrees of freedom. This, combined with X-ray imaging in real time, allows sub-millimeter accuracy. This precision results in improving the protection of OAR. It therefore allows increasing the dose per fraction and thus reduces the number of sessions (hypofractionation), with the prospect of dose escalation studies. Moreover, hypofractionation reduces the number of moves, increasing the comfort of the patient. Finally, unlike the conventional radiosurgery, the accuracy of the image guidance system eliminates the constraint of a rigid invasive stereotactic frame, imposing a single fraction.

Introduction

The development in the imaging world, being able to deliver imaging with a hundred of microns resolution, has naturally led to the need for increased precision in the therapeutic world. Reaching the sub-millimeter accuracy is often needed for radiation treatment, paving the way to introducing robots in the medical environment. Robots are widely used in many industries where precision and accuracy are necessary, so it is very logical to find them in the medical community. Stereotactic treatments aim at delivering to the patient a high dose in fewer fractions. This therapeutic solution comes with its own challenges to be overcome by the technology, such as the high dose conformality to spare healthy tissue with such a high dose delivered and intra-fraction motion management capability. To take over those challenges, the CyberKnife (Figure 1) system has been developed with unique dedicated features for the treatment, with high doses to moving or static targets anywhere in the body. The CyberKnife system uses two robots, one holding the linear accelerator, source of the X rays, and the other one driving the treatment couch. This system can be divided in four different parts: the radiation delivery system, the imaging system (X-ray tubes and receivers), the respiratory monitoring system and the tracking algorithms. Originally developed for radiosurgery, its evolution enables stereotactic treatment for the entire body, making it a standard for stereotactic treatments.

Equipment and Treatment Room

The power supply of the CyberKnife system is located in the equipment room located close to the treatment delivery room. The equipment room is composed with a PDU, generators for the X-ray imaging system, a chiller, a modulator control chassis and the robot controller. The main computer is located near the treatment room. The patient database is a common file that stores calculations and treatment; it is situated in the main computer. The control room holds several screens, which are used to display the:

- Treatment control,
- Synchrony system,
- Different cameras in the treatment room.

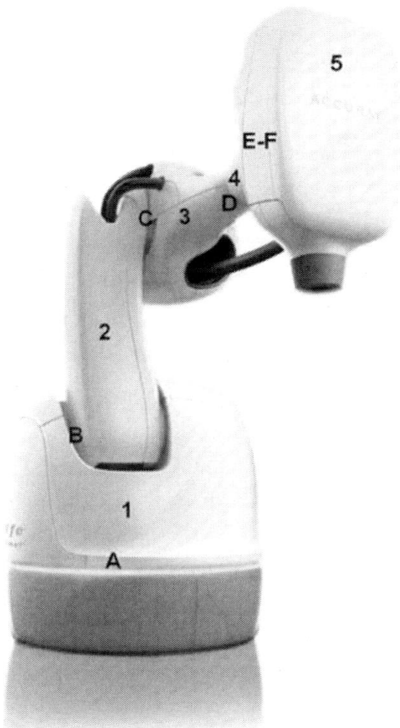

Figure 1. The CyberKnife robot (last generation).

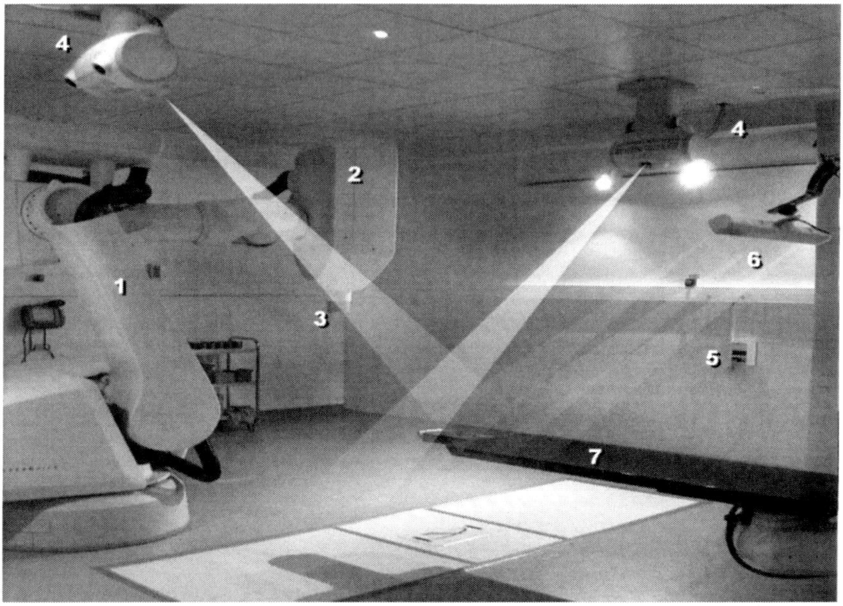

Figure 2. The CyberKnife and its suite: 1 robot, 2 accelerator, 3 collimator, 4 (2) x-ray tubes, 5 position lasers, 6 "Synchrony" camera, 7 treatment couch.

The Robot

The first machine was developed in the 1990s at Stanford University Medical Center (United States) under the direction of John R. Adler mainly for SRS purposes. Since then, the system has changed. The latest version is presented on the Figure 1 and can be compared to the previous generation, Figure 2. The simple design of the CyberKnife system remains a compact Linac, mounted onto a robotic arm (manufactured by KUKA Robotics). On the latest version (Figure1) the robotic arm used is slightly different from the previous generation, in order to allow heavier load such as the InCise collimation capability - Multi Leaf Collimator (MLC). The robotic manipulator can move in the 3D dimension, allowing rotational and translational movement of the Linac in a virtual sphere around the patient. Due to the imaging capacities that must remain available all along the treatment, the positions of the manipulator have been reduced, limiting the posterior direction to 22 degrees below the horizontal. The virtual sphere of possible positions of the Linac is divided in discrete points (295) where the manipulator will stop. Those positions are known as the "nodes" which will effectively correspond to the source position. From each of these nodes, the Linac can take 12 different beam's directions per collimator used. The total of possible beam could then be enormous also it has been limited to 6000. In order to visualize the treatment beam direction, a laser has been mounted inside the treatment head. When the robot is in rest position, the vertical axis can be verified through a reference point that is fixed to the ground ensuring that the robot calibration is accurate. The robot speed is greater than 80 degrees per second depending on the axis of rotation considered, which is equivalent to a speed up to 180 cm/s. For patient safety purposes and in order to avoid collisions or to frighten the patient, the speed has been decreased to 5% of its capacities (6-10 cm/s).

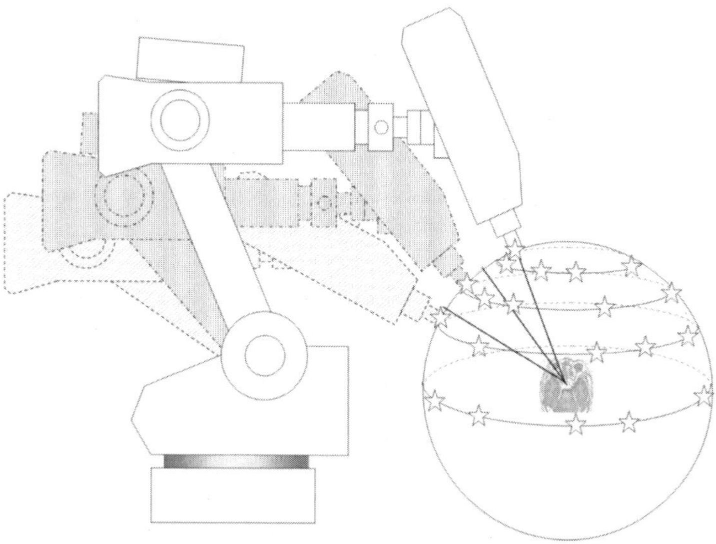

Figure 3. Example of node sets, and movement of the Cyberknife on a virtual sphere centered by the lesion.

The Collimation System

The collimation system is adapted automatically by the manipulator to the end of the Linac. The collimation systems are located on the exchange table and picked by the manipulator as needed during the treatment. The collimation system on the CyberKnife system is composed of three different types of interchangeable collimators: Fixed collimator, IRIS (Variable Aperture Collimator) and MLC.

The fixed collimators are made of tungsten copper and nickel with a fixed circular aperture. There are 12 different diameters available for treatment: 5, 7.5, 10, 12.5, 15, 20, 25, 30, 35, 40, 50, and 60 mm (Figure 4). On the new CyberKnife system, the collimators are located on the side of the exchange table and have the same height, to be differentiated from the previous system where the weight of each collimator was maintained constant, resulting in a change in collimator height (the taller for the one with the larger diameter). During the course of a treatment, up to 3 fixed collimators can be selected and will be automatically exchanged during the treatment.

The IRIS collimator (Figure 5), designed in collaboration with the DKFZ in Heidelberg, Germany, has a variable circular aperture. It is actually composed with 2 banks of 6 tungsten blocks forming a dodecagon. Theoretically the IRIS collimator can take any diameter but has been limited to those of the same discrete distribution as the fixed collimation.

The MLC system has been introduced in the latest version of the CyberKnife system. It allows random shape apertures up to 10 x 12 cm wide at the calibration distance. It is composed with 41 interdigitated leaves, 2.5 mm thick. Using the MLC the dose is delivered in a step and shoot mode, where the leaves are set in motion to the required position, then the beam is turned on.

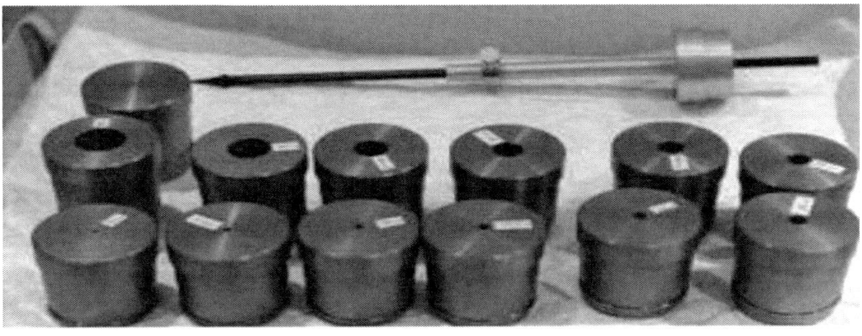

Figure 4. The collimators.

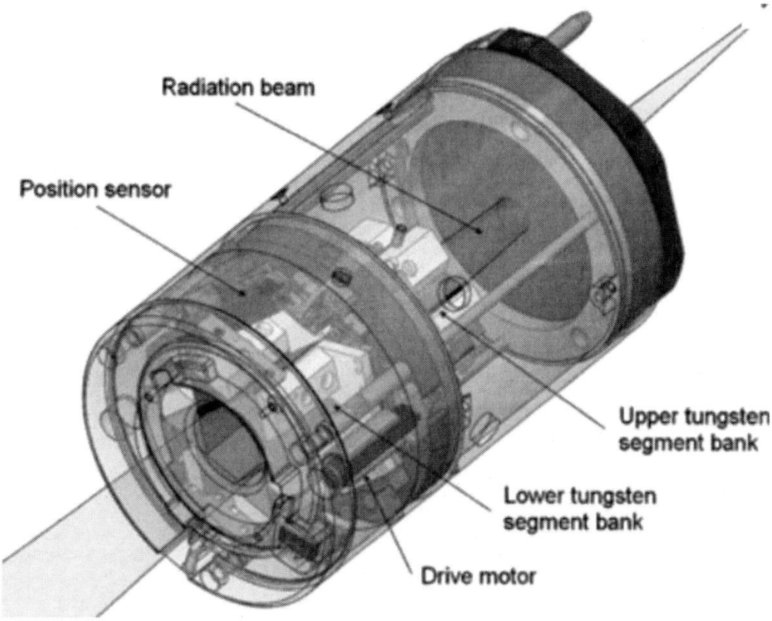

Figure 5. Iris collimator.

Characteristics of the Accelerator and the Beam

The linear accelerator mounted on the Cyberknife system's manipulator is a compact Linac producing a 6 Megavolt (MV) X-ray beam. The electrons are accelerated in the accelerating waveguide and sent directly to a tungsten target for X-ray generation without bending magnet. The X- rays are generated up to a dose rate of 1000 Monitor Units per minute (MU/Min). As for the 6 MV beams, the maximum depth is located at 15mm. The X-ray calibration is performed in a phantom to obtain 1cGy for 1 MU delivered with the largest fixed collimator (60 mm) at a distance of 800 mm from the source. The source axis distance (SAD) for treatments is between 650 and 1000 mm. The commissioning of the 6 MV X ray beam is performed by measuring the tissue maximum ratio (TMR), as seen in Figure 6, the off center ratio (OCR), as seen in Figure 7, and the output factor (OF) for the different collimation systems available.

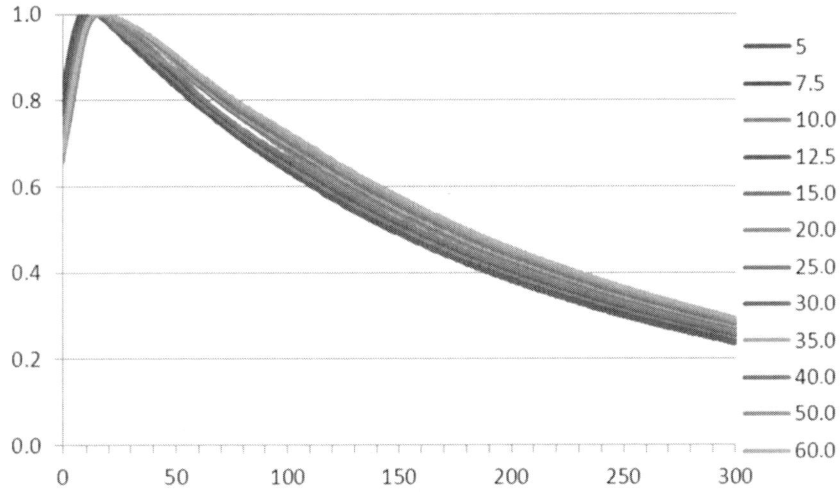

Figure 6. The depth doses for all collimators.

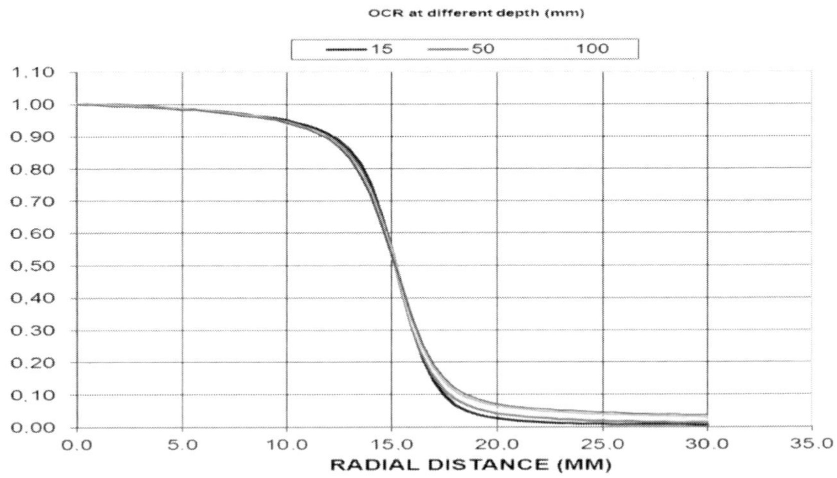

Figure 7. The off-center ratio (OCR) at different depths for the collimator with a diameter of 30 mm.

The Treatment Couch

The treatment couch is made of carbon fiber and has a narrower portion for the robot's head (allowing for a shorter travel distance). There are three translational movements (superior-inferior, anterior-posterior, and right-left) and three rotational motions (roll, pitch, and yaw). All of these movements can be controlled from the control room (which is located outside the treatment room).

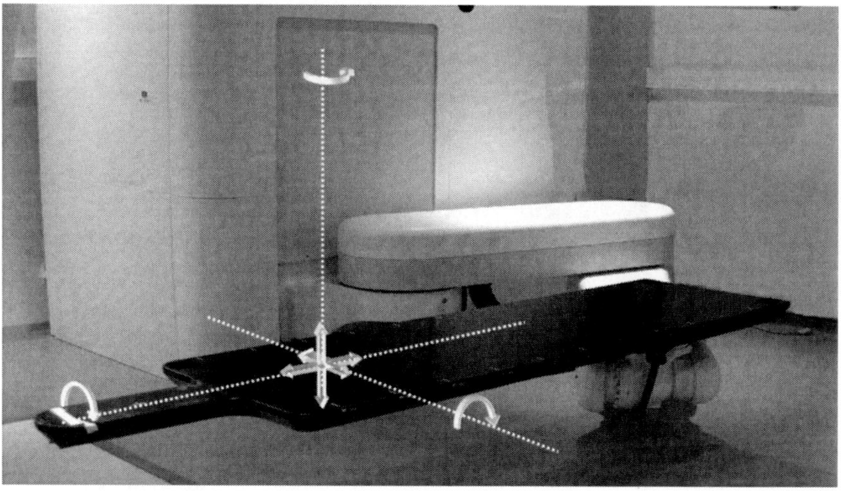

Figure 8. The treatment couch with a representation of its options for translational and rotational movements.

The Imaging System

The CyberKnife imaging system can be seen in Figure 2. It is composed of 2 X-ray sources mounted on the ceiling at 45 degrees from the vertical, thus forming a 90° angle between the central axis of each of the X-ray tubes. X-ray generators are located in the equipment room (40-125 kV; 25-300 mA). The X-ray energy can be varied up to 150 kVp depending on the depth of the target to be localized. The intersection of the 2 X-ray tubes is called the align center, even if the CyberKnife system does not have an isocenter per se, the align center is an important point of reference. Opposite to the X-ray tube, built in the floor, the cesium iodide scintillators are deposited on the amorphous Silicon photodiode detectors. The new detectors, available in the new CyberKnife generation, are composed of 1536x1536 pixels with a 0.27x0.27mm pixel size, giving a 427x427mm sensitive area, it gives a 18x18 cm field of view at the align center.

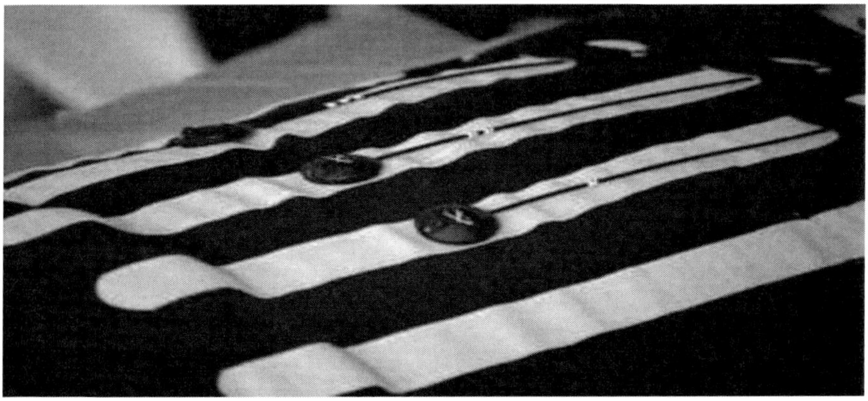

Figure 9. LED and shirt used for CyberKnife treatments with Synchrony.

The Respiratory Tracking System "Synchrony"

The CyberKnife system is known for its real time tracking capacities. The Synchrony system is a combination of a tracking algorithm and hardware responsible to follow target respiratory induced motion. The Synchrony system combines information obtained by the stereotactic cameras and the live X-ray images. The stereotactic cameras (number 6 on Figure 2) enable the system to get a continuous recording of the position of external markers placed on the patient surface. Those captors are Luminescent Electronic Device (LED) attached on the patient abdomen close to the treatment location thanks to a vest with black and white strips that the patient will wear during the treatment, see Figure 9. The stereotactic cameras are mounted in a boom bar, on the ceiling, toward the foot end of the table. Their position is adjustable in order to guaranty the optimal motion amplitude recorded during the treatment. The Synchrony system algorithm will correlate the information received from the stereotactic cameras regarding the external markers position and those received from the X ray imaging system regarding the internal markers position. This correlation enables to create a model that allows the CyberKnife system to predict the position of the target at any time during the treatment. This model representing the target position in time is sent to the manipulator to follow the target. The model is reevaluated each time a new live X-ray image pair is acquired. It can be modified, when the newly acquired internal target position falls out of the predicted model position, enabling a safe delivery and confidence that the CyberKnife system will track the real target position following the actual breathing pattern of the patient. Unexpected motion (such as coughing for example) of the patient, out of a limit tolerance set by the user, will automatically stop the beam delivery.

Safety

All of the robot's movements must be performed safely. This need for safety explains why, in addition to the touch sensor at the collimator's level, a safety volume has been created around the patient. It is designed for the two cases, the head and the body. In figure 10, the security zone for the body is represented. Cameras inside the treatment room show the movements of the robot and the couch.

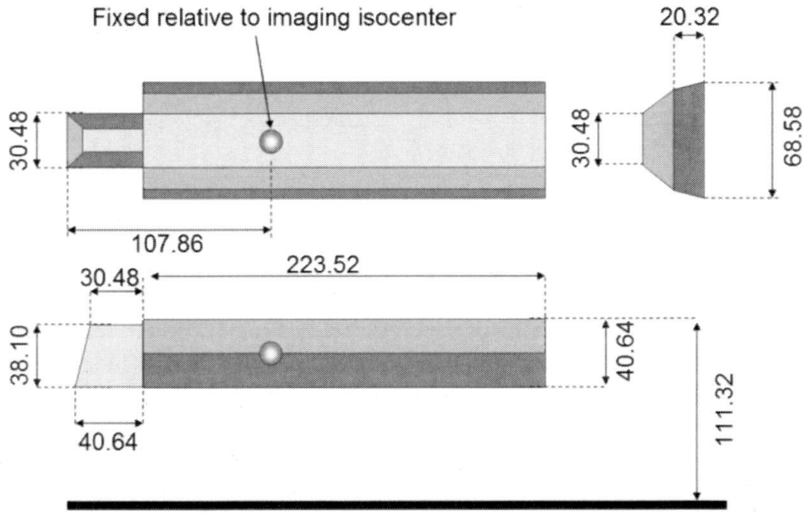

Figure 10. Fixed safety zone for body treatment.

The Software

All CyberKnife system treatments require a tracking method to be set up with regard to the localization of the target. 6 different tracking methods associated with 2 motion tracking algorithms are currently available on the CyberKnife system:

Target tracking methods:

- 6D skull tracking: allows a tracking of the skull for intracranial treatments;
- Xsight Spine: allows tracking of a spine region close to the target, taking into account the spine deformation;
- Fiducial tracking: enables to track base on fiducial implanted close to the target;
- Xsight lung: enables to locate and track directly the lung tumor;
- Lung Optimized Treatment (LOT): enables the tracking using only one X-ray image to locate and track the target;
- Xsight Prone: enables the treatment of the patient in a prone position for posterior located targets.

Motion tracking algorithms:

- Synchrony: allows building a predictive model following the respiratory induced target motion;
- In Tempo: enables to automatically detect target motion superior to a user set threshold and automatically increase the image frequency.

The different tracking methods have a similar workflow to track the target. It uses reference imaging called Digitally Reconstructed Radiograph (DRR), imported from the CT simulator. Live images taken during the treatment will be compared to those images and a registration will be performed. The offset necessary to overlay the live and DRR images will then represent the position correction. It is sent to the manipulator which moves to the planned position. The interval between live image acquisitions is determined by the therapist. This is an important factor that will define how the CyberKnife system will ensure a proper positioning of the target.

All parts of the CyberKnife (e.g., the robot, the couch and imaging system) are managed from a PC which is located in the control room. To verify the positioning of the target volume, reference images are created on the therapy planning system. Before and during treatment, images of the 2 X-ray tubes are compared to reference images. During treatment, the technician chooses the interval between images (at each beam or each set of 3 or more beams).

Before treatment, the couch is moved until there is a correspondence between the reference and X-ray images. During treatment, the couch is automatically moved to account for small changes in translation and rotation values.

Quality Control

Quality control is an important part of radiotherapy treatments, especially for the CyberKnife system with its unique tracking features. Several periodical tests are performed to ensure a correct calibration of the system. Those tests are performed daily, monthly or yearly:

- The manipulator absolute position (daily),
- The X-ray beam parameters (daily),
- The couch parameters (daily monitoring of flatness),
- The isocenter of the imaging system (monthly).

To test these parameters, different devices, called "phantoms" are delivered with the CyberKnife system (Figure 11):

- AQA phantom (Automatic Quality Assurance): a cube with a high density sphere embedded in its center. This phantom allows performing the so called Winston-Lutz test which verifies the angle position accuracy of the Linac by determining the relative offset between the halo of the sphere and the actual beam center visible on a radiochromic films after irradiation. This irradiation is performed at 0 and 90 degrees on a daily basis.
- A head phantom with 2 different inserts located in the head region and close to the spine, where radiochromic films measurement can be taken. The purpose of this phantom is to perform an End to End (E2E) test, and to use the head phantom as a real patient. The measurement obtained with the radiochromic films will be compared to the calculated values obtained via the treatment planning system.
- Synchrony phantom to test the Synchrony software for tracking respiration induced motion. The moving phantom is simulating a patient's breathing cycle. Radiochromic films are used to measure the

delivered dose that will be compared to the one calculated by the planning system.

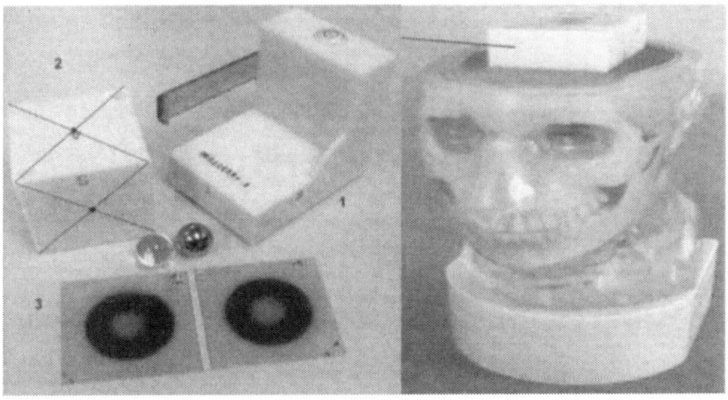

Figure 11. Left: The ball cube with radiochromic films. Right: The head phantom.

Part IIb: Tracking

In: The Revolution of Robotic …
Editor: Pierre-Yves Bondiau
ISBN: 978-1-62808-718-5

Chapter 7

CyberKnife Tracking Methods

Pierre-Yves Bondiau*
Department of Radiation Oncology,
Antoine-Lacassagne Cancer Center, Nice, France
University of Nice Sophia-Antipolis, Nice, France

Abstract

Stereotactic body radiation therapy (SBRT) is increasingly being used to treat lung cancer. SBRT delivery of high-precision irradiation is achieved by its dramatic reduction of the margins surrounding the tumor volume. Methods that are available to reduce these margins include respiratory gating, the use of a body frame, and real-time tumor tracking. Additionally, with the movement capabilities of CyberKnife, it is possible to track real-time tumor movement during the patient's breathing. Some tumors can also be tracked using image contrasts, while other tumors require that one or more fiducials be implanted into the tumor volume or its vicinity. The next two chapters in this book will present results using the following two methods:

- Contrast-based tracking method (Xsight® Lung Tracking System)
- Fiducial tracking (fiducials are usually introduced using either a computed tomography (CT) scan or bronchoscopy)

* Email: pierre-yves.bondiau@nice.unicancer.fr.

Tumors can also be treated without being tracked. In these cases, the location of the tumor is fixed and its surrounding margins are increased in order to accommodate the tumor's movements during the patient's breathing. One way to fix a tumor is to use the spine to localize the lung's upper lobe.

Lung Treatment Methods

1) Overview of Tumor Tracking Methods

We treat lung tumors in four different ways. First, if the tumor does not move while the patient is breathing, we use the Xsight® Spine Tracking System (Accuray Incorporated, Sunnyvale, California, USA) (XSP). This software allows us to treat a tumor near (≤ 3 cm) a bone structure such as the spine. Second, if the tumor moves while the patient is breathing, we use the Synchrony® Respiratory Motion Tracking System software. This software synchronizes the movements of the CyberKnife robot with the movements of the patient's breathing. Third, the location of the tumor during the patient's breathing can be detected either by locating the fiducial that is inserted within the tumor or by using the contrast-based method of the Xsight Lung Tracking System (XLTS).

Defining which tracking method to use is very important. If the XLTS method is possible or if the tumor doesn't move with the patient's breathing (see Figures 1 and 2), the dosimetric CT scan or the dosimetric PET scan (see annex D) can be done immediately. However, if the XLTS method cannot be used and the tumor does move with the patient's breathing, a fiducial needs to be inserted into the tumor. Depending on the tumor's location, this fiducial insertion can be done using a CT scan or fibroscopy.

2) Contrast-Based Tracking Method (XLTS)

XLTS is a method that directly tracks soft tissue during respiratory motion. Invasive fiducial implantation procedures are thus not needed, thereby decreasing the patient's time to treatment and eliminating the risk of pneumothorax and other fiducial placement complications. Direct tumor tracking can be performed for visible tumors by registering the tumor region in digitally reconstructed radiographs (DRRs), generated from the planning CT image, to the corresponding region in the treatment X-ray images. Image processing is used to enhance the visibility of the lung tumor in the DRRs and X-ray images.

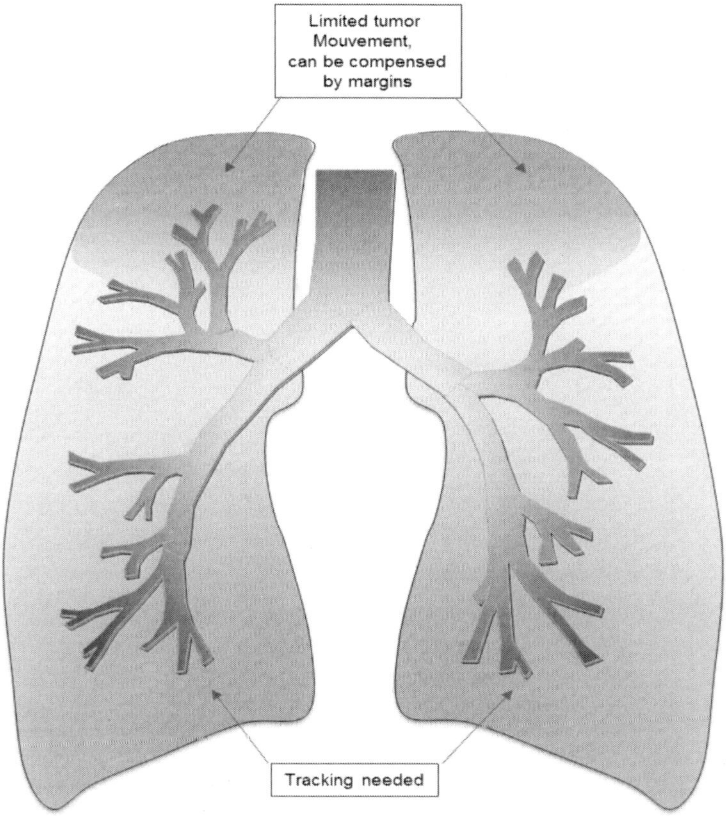

Figure 1. If XLTS or fiducials cannot be used, the movement of the tumor into the upper lobe can be compensated for by the addition of tissue margins (see annex B). To avoid the use of overly large margins, fiducial/tumor tracking may be necessary.

In most cases, a tumor with a diameter of > 1.5 cm can be tracked using the contrast-based tumor tracking method that is available with XLTS. Depending on the position of the tumor, the X-ray images can potentially reveal at least one of the tumor's projections (see Figure 3). Although more robust results are given when the XLTS software is provided with 2 projections, it can also function with just 1 projection.

However, if the 45° projection of the tumor is located on the spine, the contrast between the lung and the tumor will be lost in the high level contrast of the vertebra (see Figure 4). Results arising from the use of XLTS will be presented in chapter 2.3.3.

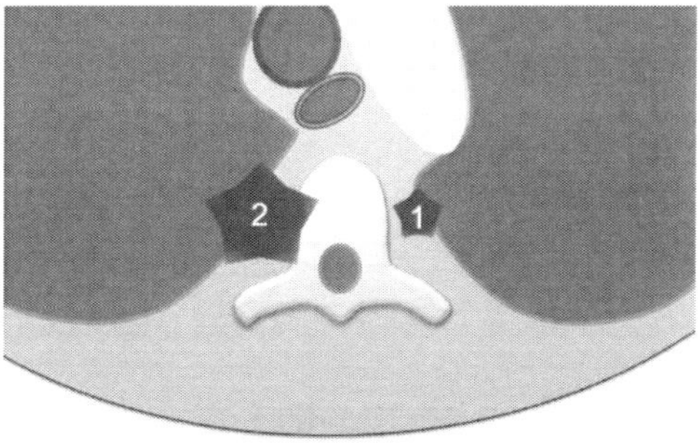

Figure 2. A paraspinal (1) or vertebra-invading tumor (2) is not affected by breathing movement; tracking is therefore not needed.

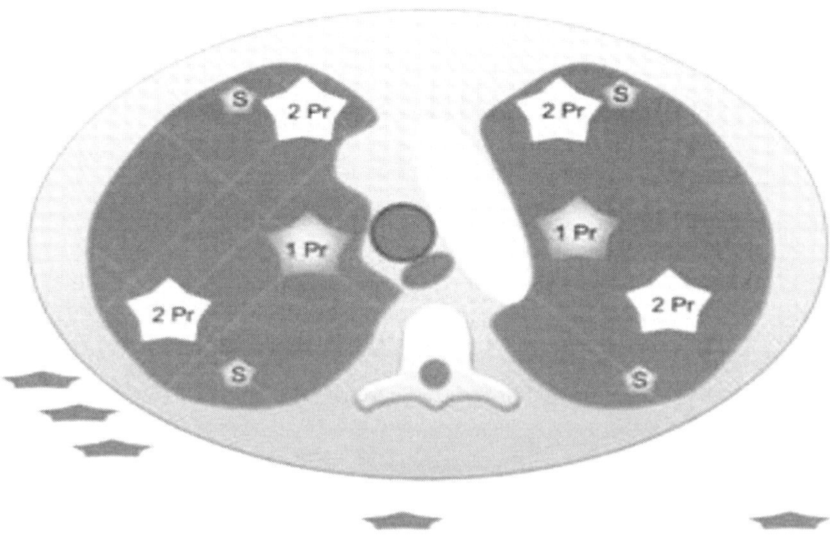

Figure 3. Tumor localization and contrast-based tumor tracking. S: A tumor that is too small for contrast-based tracking; 1 Pr: A location where it is possibile to track a tumor with 1 projection; 2 Pr: tumor tracking with 2 projections.

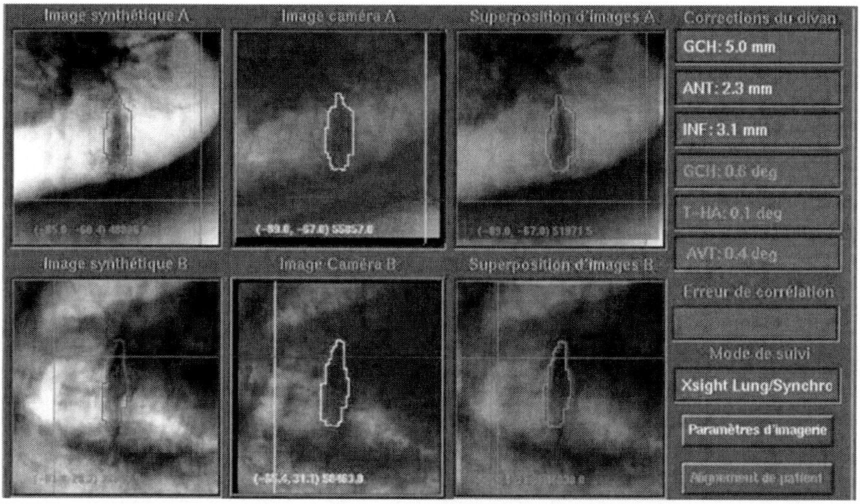

Figure 4. Automatic localization of a tumor using a contrast-based algorithm (left and middle columns) and its correction (right column).

3) Fiducial-Based Tracking Method

If a tumor has a diameter of < 1.5 cm or a poor contrast level, it is necessary to use fiducials. Depending on the treatment team, 1 or 3 or more fiducials can be implanted.

The implantation of 1 fiducial enables only the tracking of translation, whereas the insertion of 3 or more fiducials allows for the tracking of both translation and rotation. Depending on the location of the tumor, fiducials can be inserted using a CT scan or fibroscopy. The advantages and convenience of fiducial insertion via fibroscopy will be presented in Chapter 2.3.2.

However, the use of fiducials increases the patient's required time to treatment, possible pain, and the risk of complications, the most significant of which is pneumothorax (see Figure 5).

The risk of pneumothorax occurs in 5-15% of treated patients and its occurrence depends on where the tumor is localized, how many fiducials were used, and the team's experience. Although less frequent than pneumothorax, fiducial migration may also occur (Figure 6). On the other hand, fiducials allow for real-time tumor tracking.

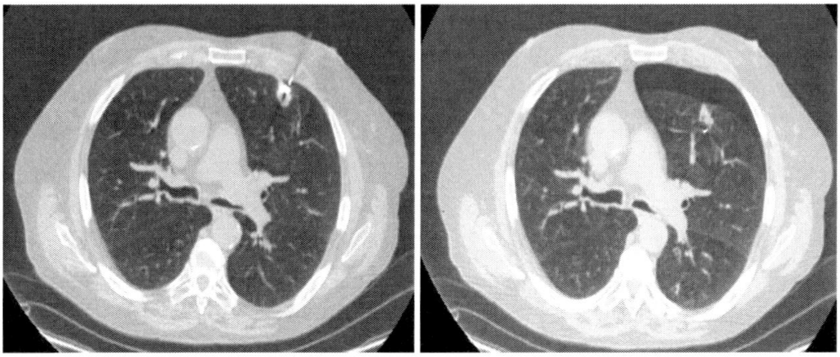

Figure 5. Left: The vertebra before fiducial insertion; Right: Pneumothorax in the vertebra after fiducial insertion.

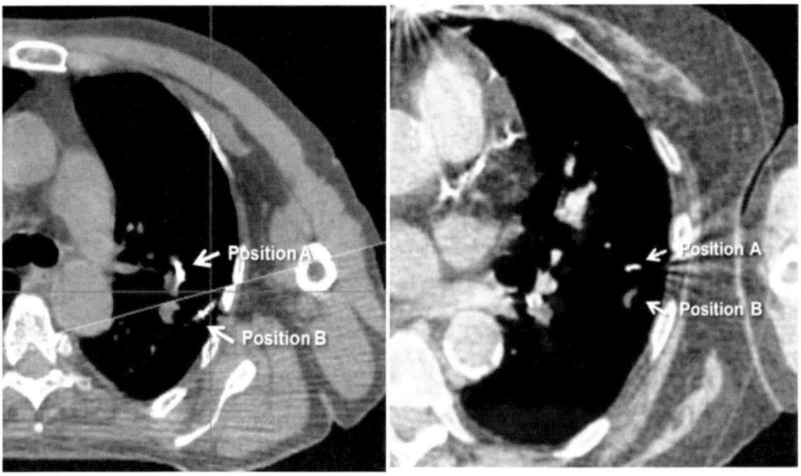

Figure 6. Left: a fused CT scan showing fiducial migration from position A to position B for patient #1; Right: a fused CT scan showing fiducial migration from position A to position B for patient #2.

4) Other Tracking Methods

Some tumors, such as those that invade the spine, do not move when the patient breathes and can be effectively treated with the detection of bones contrast, In these cases the software is named Xsight spine.

In some others cases, if fiducial insertion is not medically possible, the movement of the tumor during a patient's breathing be compensated for by an increase in the tissue margins. To learn more about the value of margins, see annex B.

Conclusion

Depending on the tumor's location in the lung, it may be possible to detect it with the use of contrast. In other cases, it is necessary to insert fiducials.

Different types of fiducials can be used, such as "golden anchor", coils...

If a tumor does not move when the patient breathes, direct bone-based contrast detection can be used.

In: The Revolution of Robotic …
Editor: Pierre-Yves Bondiau

ISBN: 978-1-62808-718-5

Chapter 8

Role of Bronchoscopy in Implantation of Fiducial Markers for CyberKnife Treatment of Pulmonary Tumors

S. Marco,[1,2] Pierre-Yves Bondiau,[3,4] C. H. Marquette[1,2] and M. Poudenx[4,2]

[1]Department of Pneumology, Thoracic Oncology and Respiratory Intensive Care, Hôpital Pasteur,
Centre Hospitalier Universitaire de Nice, France
[2]University of Nice Sophia-Antipolis, Nice, France
[3]Department of Radiation Oncology, Antoine-Lacassagne Cancer Center, Nice, France
[4]Department of Medical Oncology, Antoine-Lacassagne Cancer Center, Nice, France

Abstract

The CyberKnife® System is a stereotactic radiotherapy technique that allows treatment of pulmonary tumors found in inoperable patients. Most often, it requires implantation of fiducial markers (FM) to allow tracking of the tumor. The standard technique is performed transparietally. The current work aims to evaluate the efficacy of bronchoscopic FM implantation.

Three techniques using three different instruments are described: the bronchoscopic protected catheter brush (BPCB), Wang's transmucosal needle aspiration, and Storz rigid lymph node bronchoscopy. A chest X-ray was taken following each procedure to confirm the number of FMs in place (T0). At the time of the planning CT, another determination of the number and position of the FMs was made (T1); and just prior to the first session with CyberKnife, the final observation was entered. The efficacy of each method was determined based on the number of FMs used, compared with the number actually implanted, and the number of patients where the different method was applied.

Thirty-eight patients underwent 41 procedures to have at least one FM bronchoscopically implanted each. One to five markers were implanted per patient (mean, 2.7) for a total of 112 FMs. The effectiveness of the techniques was modest at best: 46% for all three techniques combined; 17% for BPCB; 46% for Wang's needle; and 67% for the Storz bronchoscope. Despite this, only two implantation-related treatment delays occurred, or 6%, of the patients to be treated with CyberKnife.

Endoscopy is a complimentary technique to the transparietal approach for implantation of FMs. Its effectiveness is acceptable if several FMs are placed. Storz rigid lymph node bronchoscopy appears to be the most reliable of the techniques; however, it is performed under general anaesthesia and applies only to central lesions. Wang's needle is an alternative.

Introduction

Transthoracic approach is the first technique employed by our team for FM placement. Unfortunately, it has many contraindications (pulmonary emphysema, treatment with anti-platelet drugs, coagulation disorders, and inaccessible central lesions), and a significant risk of pneumothorax (13% to 47% in different studies) [8-10].

Some teams are therefore interested in other approaches such as the vascular approach (coils), and the endoscopic approach [11, 12]. The latter does not have dedicated equipment for implantation of markers, unlike the transparietal approach. Our interventional bronchoscopy team was tapped to place one to several FM in patients with pulmonary cancer who would be treated with CyberKnife. This study describes the equipment used, and also the efficiency of this approach and its complications.

Materials and Methods

Endpoints

This prospective descriptive study was conducted between May 2007 and April 2010 at the Centre Hospitalier Universitaire de Nice in the Department of Pulmonology, Thoracic Oncology, and Intensive Care, and the Antoine Lacassagne Cancer Center in Nice.

The principal endpoint of this study is, to assess the efficiency of this technique. The latter is defined by the following parameters:

- Efficiency by FM: number of FM used during treatment / number of FM implanted
- Efficiency per patient: Number of patients treated / number of patients with intention to treat with CyberKnife.

Secondary endpoints are: complications related to placement of FMs and those related to treatment with CyberKnife, as well as efficacy of treatment according to RECIST criteria [13].

Inclusion Criteria

Inclusion criteria were a pulmonary lesion for which treatment by CyberKnife is indicated and propriety of fiducial implantation through a bronchoscopic approach.

Equipment Used

FM are sterile gold cylinders with 4-mm by 0.8-mm dimensions. Several instruments – either alone or in combination – can be used implanting FMs with an endoscopic approach, such as bronchoscopic protected catheter brush (BPCB) (Telemed Systems, Inc., ref 3102, Hudson, MA, U.S.A.), Wang's transmucosal aspiration needle (BARD Endoscopic Technologies, ref MW319, Billerica, MA, U.S.A.) [14], and Storz rigid lymph node bronchoscopy needle (Karl Storz Endoscopy –America, Inc., El Segundo, CA, U.S.A.). The choice of technique depends on the location of the lesion and the type of anesthesia to be used. The Storz needle is rigid and it can only be used for central lesions. The procedure is done using rigid bronchoscopy under general anesthesia. Wang's needle and BPCB implantations are procedures of flexible fibroscopy and can be used for central or peripheral lesions under local or general anesthesia. For central lesions, if the lesion is not visible on endoscopy, the technique is combined with endobronchial ultrasound (EBUS) (Olympus America, Inc., BF-UC160F-OL8, Center Valley, PA, U.S.A.). For peripheral lesions, electromagnetic navigation bronchoscopy (ENB) (superDimension, Inc., Minneapolis, MN, U.S.A.) can orient the surgeon by locating the tumor.

Data Collection

Data collection concerned clinical characteristics of patients such as age, sex, medical history (especially respiratory, cardiovascular, and neoplastic), performance status (PS) [15], and Charlson comorbidity index [16]. The characteristics of the treated tumor were noted such as its location, TNM classification and stage [1], and prior treatments. We defined central lesions as any lesion accessible by flexible fibroscopy, and peripheral lesions as any non-central lesion. The number of FM implanted, the technique employed, and the adverse events and complications were noted. After the implantation, the following steps were defined:

- T0: four hours after implantation, AP and lateral chest X-rays were taken;
- T1: during planning CT;
- T2: right before the treatment.

At each step, the number of FM was noted, as well as the number of FM used for tracking. The doses received by the patient and the immediate and late complications corresponding to these doses were recorded. The local tumor response at six months according to RECIST criteria was also collected [13].

Statistical Study

Due to the limited number of patients enrolled in the study, no statistical studies were undertaken.

Results

Patients and Tumors Treated

The study was conducted from May 2007 to May 2010. Forty-one procedures to implant FM were performed on 38 patients; three patients underwent a second procedure. Table 1 summarizes the clinical characteristics of the patients. Mean age was 67.5 years (range, 47–82 years) and the cohort consisted of 24 men and 14 women. The PS was 0 in 58% of patients, 1 in 37%, and 2 in 5%. Mean Charlson index was 5.6 (range, 3–9). Most patients smoked or had smoked, which may explain the significant number of respiratory and cardiovascular comorbidities. Thirty-five percent of patients had a previous history of cancer different from current disease, including 21% bronchopulmonary cancer. We had performed three pneumonectomies, three lobectomies, and two segmentectomies.

Most patients were treated with CyberKnife for a localized inoperable lung tumor (58%), including 16% for a recurrence of NCBSC or a pulmonary metastasis. Majority of patients – 68% – had NSCLC. Note that in 21%, the neoplastic origin of the lesion could not be proven histologically, but was shown by an increased uptake in PET-CT and/or an increase in size over two thoracic CT scans at three- or six-month intervals. 66% of the lesions were centrally located and 33% were peripheral. Table 2 summarizes tumor characteristics.

Equipment

The procedure was conducted under general anesthesia in 78% (32/41) despite the patients' comorbidities. Local anesthesia was preferred in cases of contraindication to general anesthesia and/or for central lesions. One hundred twelve FMs were placed; 65% (73/112) by Wang needle, 19% (21/112) by Storz needle, and 16% (18/112) by BPCB. In one patient, the implantation was not possible because the segmental bronchus to be catheterized was not accessible through flexible endoscopy.

The Wang needle consists of a catheter and two needles, one external (histology needle) and one internal (cytology needle). The FM placed in the external needle is pushed into the lesion through the internal needle (Figure 1). A few adverse events associated with the Wang needle were noted: five FM were lost in the tracheo-bronchial tree and two fibroscopes were damaged during Wang needle procedures. When removed, the external needle was too far from the distal reinforcement zone. This resulted in a tear in the sheath of the operating channel of the fibroscope when it was bent.

Table 1. Clinical characteristics of patients in our series

				interval
Age (years)	Mean	67.5		47-82
PS	0	58%	(22/38)	
	1	37%	(14/38)	
	2	5%	(2/38)	
Charlson Index	mean	5.6		3-9
	≤ 5	34%	(13/38)	
	> 5	66%	(25/38)	
History				
Cardiovascular		45%	(17/38)	
	MI	18%	(7/38)	
	CAF	21%	(8/38)	
	arteriopathy	7%	(3/38)	
Respiratory		29%	(11/38)	
Other cancer:		35%	(13/38)	
	Lung	21%	(8/38)	
	Prostate	5%	(2/38)	
	ENT	3%	(1/38)	
	Testicular	3%	(1/38)	
	Breast	3%	(1/38)	

Legend: *"PS"*: performance status; *"MI"*: myocardial infarction; "*CAF*": chronic atrial fibrillation

Table 2. Characteristics of pulmonary tumors in our series

Indications for CyberKnife treatment	Inoperable localized pulmonary tumor	58%	(22/38)
	Recurrence of NSCBC	16%	(6/38)
	Non-resectable pulmonary metastasis	16%	(6/38)
	Patient refusal of surgery	10%	(4/38)

Localized treatment-naïve pulmonary tumors	IA		32%	(12/38)
	IB		26%	(10/38)
	IIA		5%	(2/38)
	IIB		3%	(1/38)
	IIIA		3%	(1/38)
Histology	NSCBC		68%	(26/38)
		Bronchial ADK	35%	(13/38)
		Bronchial SC	24%	(9/38)
	Pulmonary metastases from a known primary		10%	(4/38)
		Renal	5%	(2/38)
		Colon	3%	(1/38)
		Uterine	3%	(1/38)
	No histology		21%	(8/38)
Location	Central		68%	(26/38)
	Peripheral		32%	(12/38)

Legend: "*NSCBC*": non-small cell bronchial carcinoma; "*ADK*": adenocarcinoma; "*SC*": squamous cell carcinoma.

Figure 1 displays a patient course before treatment with CyberKnife®. FM implantation was done during bronchial fibroscopy under general anesthesia with diagnostic electromagnetic navigation. Access being difficult, the implantation of FM was then decided, even though a treatment with CyberKnife® had not been discussed by the multidisciplinary panel. Finally, CyberKnife® treatment was not selected by the original multidisciplinary panel.

The BPCB consists of a catheter, inside which the FM is placed, upstream from a brush. When the operator is in position, such as a tumoral stenosis or a friable tumor, the brush pushes the FM out.

The technique using the Storz needle has never been described in the literature, and was developed by our team. It requires a central venous catheter (CVC) to push the FM, and is conducted using rigid bronchoscopy under general anesthesia. When the needle is implanted in or near the mucosa under visual control, the FM is slid in the needle and pushed through the CVC (Figure 2).

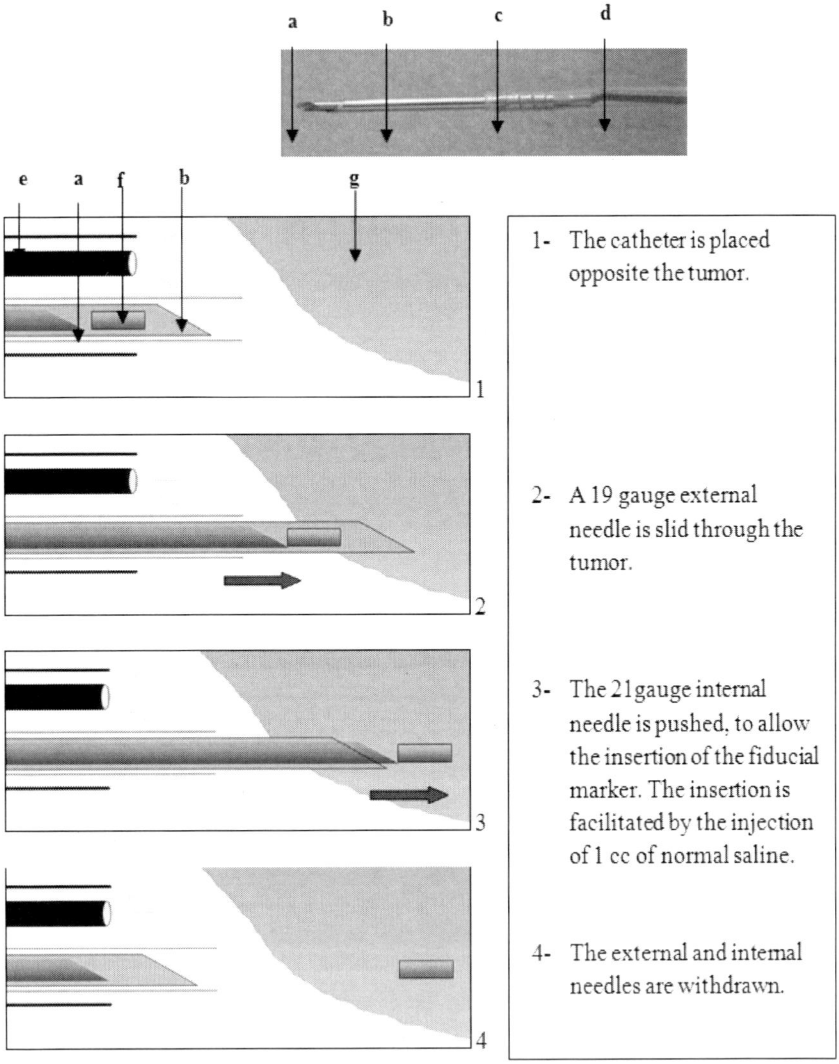

Legend: (A) internal needle, (B) external needle, (C) catheter reinforcement area, (D) Wang needle catheter (E) flexible fibroscope, (F) fiducial marker, (G) bronchial tumor.

Figure 1. insertion of fiducial markers through the Wang needle.

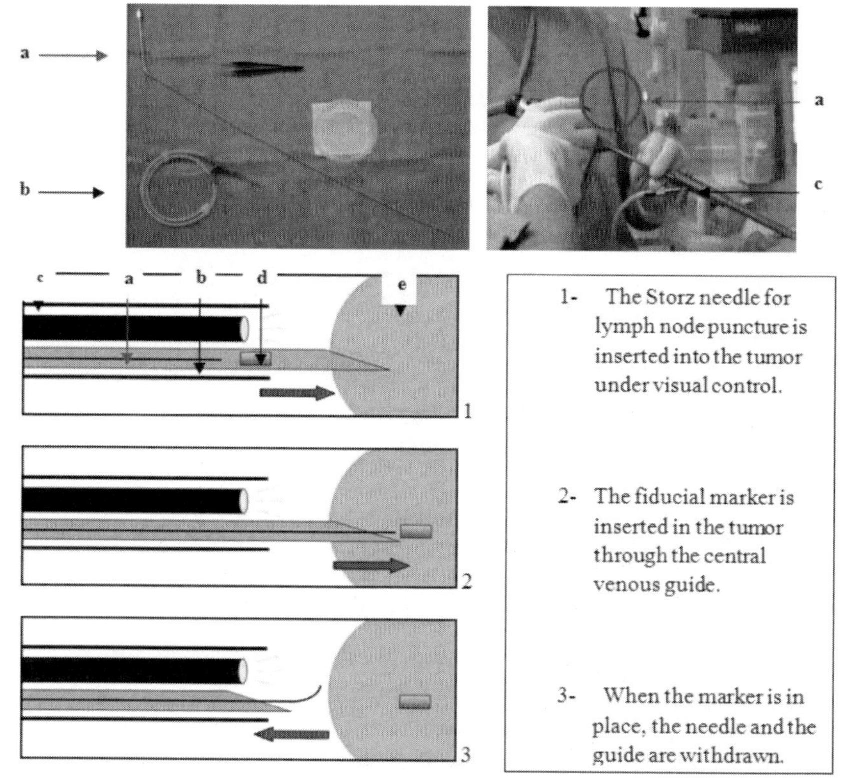

Legend: (A) Storz needle, (B) central venous catheter, (C) rigid bronchoscopy tube, (D): fiducial marker, (E): bronchial tumor.

Figure 2. Insertion of fiducial markers through the Storz needle for lymph node puncture.

Efficiency

We assessed the efficiency of each method by determining the number of FM present in the relevant area during different stages of the treatment process. Figure 3 shows the patients' progress through this process. In one patient, no FMs were found during the planning CT. Given the presence of severe comorbidities (pneumonectomy with NSCBC, a recent MI, clopidogrel prescription, with active alcohol and tobacco use), it was decided that another procedure for FM placement would not be attempted. Among the 32 patients who were treated before the end of April 2010, 63% of FMs were still present in the lungs, and 46% of FM were utilized in tracking. Two patients did not receive treatment with CyberKnife after FM placement. One patient was canceled due to the onset of brain metastases before the planning CT study, and the second after a reconsideration of the patient's file by the original multidisciplinary panel. Two patients were not yet treated at the time of analysis. 94% of the patients had completed their treatment at the time of this work. Table 3 summarizes the number of FM present and the number of FM used to track the tumor, as a result of each technique employed. The efficacy of the Storz needle seems to be the best of the three at 67%. This technique requires general anesthesia and is utilized only for central lesions. The Wang needle technique was found to have an efficiency of 48-49%. This technique is most appropriate for patients with peripheral lesions or a contraindication to general anesthesia (Table 4). The efficacy of the Storz catheter is poor: used alone, its efficiency is 17%; used in comb, it decreases the efficiency of other techniques.

Complications Secondary to Implanting FM

Immediate complications related to FM implantation were the following: minimal bleeding (five patients), bronchospasm responsive to aerosol therapy (two patients), and symptomatic complete pneumothorax drained by a Fuhrman drain (one patient). It should be noted that a few weeks after the placement of FMs, one patient had infective endocarditis with cerebral embolism, in the context of a known valvulopathy. There is no evidence that the implantation of FM was linked to this infection.

Treatment and Response

Thirty-two patients were treated with CyberKnife before the end of April 2010. We define the gross tumor volume (GTV) as the macroscopic tumoral volume delineated in mediastinum windowing. Clinical tumor volume is define as GTV with a 5 mm margin. Planified tumor volume is the CTV with 1 mm margin. The doses received were 3 fractions of 20 Gy for peripheral lesions, and 5 fractions from 9 Gy to 15 Gy for central lesions, depending of clinical case (re-irradiation,…). Complications related to treatment were minor events such as one bronchial exacerbation in a patient with obstructive bronchopneumopathy and two asymptomatic radiation-induced pneumopathies.

Table 3. Efficacy of FM implantation according to different techniques and tumor location

		BPCB catheter	**Wang needle**	**Storz needle**	**BPCB catheter + Wang needle**	**BPCB catheter + Storz needle**	**Total**
FM present at T2	All locations	33% (2/6)	62% (36/56)	73% (11/15)	54% (7/13)	70% (7/10)	63% (63/100)
FM used at T2	All locations	17% (1/6)	46% (26/56)	67% (10/15)	23% (3/13)	60% (6/10)	46% (46/100)
	Central lesions	-	49% (13/29)	67% (10/15)	23% (3/13)	60% (6/10)	48% (32/67)
	Peripheral lesions	17% (1/6)	48% (13/27)	-	-	-	42% (14/33)

Table 4. Literature review on the efficiency and complications of endoscopically implanted FM

Authors	Number of patients	Tools	Efficiency	Complications
Harada et al. [14]	18	Catheter + hard plastic guide	65%	
Imura et al. [20]	32	"?" + ENB	75%	Partial pneumothorax non-drained (1 patient)
Reichner et al. [21]	18	Wang needle	78%	Embolization of a subsegmental artery of the pulmonary artery (3 FM) Bronchospasm with 48h IOT(1 patient)
Anantham et al. [24]	57	DPB catheter + ENB	89%	Exacerbation of COPD at 24 hours (1 patient)
Harley et al. [23]	43	DPB catheter or Wang needle + ENB or EBUS	90.6%	Drained pneumothorax (1 patient)

Legend: Efficiency: number of patients treated / total number of patients, ENB: electro-magnetic navigation, EBUS: endobronchial ultrasound.

Nineteen patients were evaluable at six months. 13 patients were unevaluable for the following reasons: two had died, one from a pulmonary embolism at one month, the second of disease progression at five months; in two patients, due to radiation-induced pneumopathy, the diameter of the lesion was not measurable; the results of the re-evaluation at six months were not available for one patient; and eight patients had not yet reached six-month follow-up. Response to the treatment was poor: 5% (one patient) had complete response (CR), 16% (three patients) had partial response, 32% (six patients) had stable disease, and 47% had distant or local progressive disease (9 patients). Median survival was 10 months during a follow-up of one to 22 months.

Discussion

The patient cohort was heterogeneous, with some in an advanced stages of their disease. Three patients had stage II disease, one patient had stage one disease, six patients were experiencing pulmonary recurrences, and six patients' tumors were metastatic. Additionally, the patients presented with severe comorbidities. It is probably for these reasons that the response to treatment was not at the level we were hoping. According to Van der Voort van Zyp et al. [17], survival at six months is greater than 80% for patients with a Charlson index between 1 and 4.

Implanting fiducial markers endoscopically is a rare technique [12, 17-22] (Table 4). Harada's team was the first to use endoscopy placing spherical FMs through a polytetrafluoroethylene catheter [12]. Efficiency was moderate, with a rate of 65% of treated patients. Over time, techniques have improved [18-20] with increasing use of echo-endoscopy [21] and ENB [21, 22] to guide operators. Harley et al., was able to treat 90.6% of the patients successfully after endoscopic FM [21]

Our results show the Storz needle appears to be the most effective tool for central lesions. Additionally, he Wang needle can be used for patients with contraindications to general anesthesia. These two techniques may be combined with EBUS. For peripheral lesions, the Wang needle is preferred and can be combined with ENB, if necessary. The BPCB does not appear to be a reliable enough tool for this purpose as a first choice.

The standard approach is the transthoracic approach, with an efficiency allowing treatment in 91% of patients [12], with a mean of 1.05 FM placed/patient. However, this technique has a high risk of pneumothorax and multiple contraindications, in particular, inaccessible lesions (more central), and patients with severe pulmonary emphysema increase the risk of complications [8, 10]. Moreover, it is these patients who are subject to the endoscopic approach. Consequently, these two placement techniques (transthoracic and endoscopic) are not indicated for the same patients, and are therefore complementary.

Complications related to the placement of FM by endoscopy are rare and acceptable (Table 4). Still to be answered is the question of the role of prophylactic antibiotics in patients with an elevated risk of infective endocarditis.

At the start of the study, it was thought that this technique would enable us to correctly place at least three FM, enabling us to account for the rotations of the tumor during tracking. In our series, this was possible in only three patients. Placement of several FMs leads to a reduced risk of failure. Haley et al., showed that at least three FMs should be implanted for central lesions and four to five for peripheral lesions.

Conclusion

The placement of FM endoscopically is feasible, with a low and acceptable risk of complications. The efficiency of this approach is comparable to the transthoracic approach, if several FM are placed (between three and five), and if a repeat attempt is made in case of initial failure. However, this system has some limitations, and the placement of FM remains mandatory in certain cases.

References

[1] The International Association for the Study of Lung Cancer lung cancer *J Thorac Oncol*. 2007 Dec;2(12):1067-77.

[2] Massard G. Critères de qualité de la chirurgie d'exérèse des cancers bronchiques non microcellulaires. *Rev Mal Respir* 2007 ; 24 : 6S40-9.

[3] Motohiro A, Ueda H, Komatsu H, et al. Prognosis of non-surgically treated, clinical stage I lung cancer patients in Japan. *Lung Cancer* 2002; 36 : 65-9.

[4] Qiao X, Tullgren O, Lax I, et al. The role of radiotherapy in treatment of stage I non-small cell lung cancer. *Lung Cancer*, 2003 ; 41(4)1-1.

[5] Dupuy DE, Zagoria RJ, Akerley W, et al. Percutaneous radiofrequency ablation of malignancies in the lung. *AJR Am J Roentgenol.* 2000 Jan; 174(1):57-9.

[6] Uematsu M, Shioda A, Tahara K, et al. Focal, high dose, and fractionated modified stereotactic radiation therapy for lung carcinoma patients. A preliminary experience. *Cancer* 1998;82:1062–70.

[7] Muacevic A, Drexler C, Wowra B, et al. Technical description, phantom, accuracy and clinical feasibility for single-session lung radiosurgery using robotic image-guided real-time respiratory tumor tracking. *Technol Cancer Res Treat* 2007 ; 6 (4)321-8.

[8] Manhire A, Charig M, Clelland C, et al. Guidelines for radiologically guided lung biopsy. Thorax 2003 ; 58 : 920-36.

[9] Castelli J, Thariat J, Padovani B, et al. Feasibility and efficacy of cyberknife radiotherapy for lung cancer : early results. *Cancer Radiother* 2008 ; 12 (8)793-9.

[10] Kothary N, Heit JJ, Louie JD, et al. Safety and efficacy of percutaneous fiducial marker implantation for image-guided radiation therapy. *J Vasc Interv Radiol* 2009 ; 20 : 235-9.

[11] Prevost JB, Nuyttens J, Hoogeman M, et al. Endovascular coils as lung tumour markers in real-time tumour tracking stereotactic radiotherapy : preliminary results. *Eur Radiol* 2008 ;18 : 1569-76.

[12] Harada T, Shirato H, Ogura S, et al. Real-time tumor tracking radiation therapy for lung carcinoma by the aid of insertion, of a gold marker using bronchofiberscopy. *Cancer* 2002 : 95 (8) ; 1720-7.

[13] Therasse P, Arbuck SG, Eisenhauer EA, et al. New guidelines to evaluate the response to treatment in solid tumors. European Organization for Research and Treatment of Cancer, National Cancer Institute of the United States, National Cancer Institute of Canada. *J Natl Cancer Inst* 2000 ; 92(3)205-16.

[14] Wang Ko Pen. Flexible Transbronchial Needle Aspiration Biopsy for histologic Specimens. *Chest* 1985 ; 88 : 860-3.

[15] Oken M, Creech R, Tormey D, et al. Toxicity and response criteria of the Eastern Cooperative Oncology Group. *Am J Clin Oncol* 1982 ; 5 : 649-55.

[16] Charlson ME, Pompei P, Ales KL et al. A new method of classifying comorbidity in longitudinal studies : development and validation. *J Chronic Dis* 1987 ; 40 (5)373-83.

[17] Van der Voort van Zyp NC, Prevost JB, Hoogeman MS et al. Stereotactic radiotherapy with real-time tumor tracking for non-small

cell lung cancer : clinical outcome. *Radiother Oncol* 2009 ; 91 : 296-300.

[18] Imura M, Yamazaki K, Shirato H, et al. Insertion and fixation of fiducial markers for setup and tracking of lung tumors in radiotherapy. *Int J Radiation Oncology Biol Phys* 2005 ; 63 (5): 1442-47.

[19] Reichner C, Collins B, Gagnon G, et al. The placement of gold fiducials for Cyberknife stereotactic radiosurgery using a modified transbronchial needle aspiration technique. *Journal of bronchology* 2005. 12(4)193-5.

[20] Anderson E, Collins B, Gagnon G, et al. Fiducial placement for Cyberknife stereotactic radiosurgery using flexible bronchoscopy and modified transbronchial aspiration needle technique. *Chest* 2006, Supplément ; 130 (4)147.

[21] Harley DP, Krimsky WS, Sarkar S et al. Fiducial marker placement using endobronchial ultrasound and navigational bronchoscopy for stereotactic radiosurgery: an alternative strategy. *Ann Thorac Surg* 2010; 89 : 368-374.

[22] Anantham D, Feller-Kopman D, Shanmugham LN, et al. Electromagnetic navigation bronchoscopy-guided fiducial placement for robotic stereotactic radiosurgery of lung tumor. *Chest* 2007; 132 ; 930-5.

In: The Revolution of Robotic …
Editor: Pierre-Yves Bondiau
ISBN: 978-1-62808-718-5

Chapter 9

Image-Guided Stereotactic Body Radiation Therapy with Fiducial-Free Tumor Tracking for Lung Cancer

Jean-Emmanuel Bibault*, Bernard Prevost, Eric Dansin, Xavier Mirabel, Thomas Lacornerie and Eric F. Lartigau

Department of Radiation Oncology, Oscar Lambret Cancer Center, University Lille II and ONCOLille Consortium, Lille, France

Abstract

Stereotactic body radiation therapy for early-stage lung cancer can be achieved using respiratory gating, a body frame, or real-time target and motion tracking. Two target tracking methods are currently available with the CyberKnife® Robotic Radiosurgery System. The first method, fiducial tracking, requires that radiopaque markers be implanted near or inside the tumor, while the second method, the Xsight® Lung Tracking System (XLTS) is fiducial-free. XLTS directly synchronizes its targeting of the tumor with the motion of the tumor that is due to the patient's respiration. While the use of fiducials to track tumors is well documented, the clinical relevance of tracking without fiducials has yet to be well described.

* E-mail: j-bibault@o-lambret.fr.

Patients and Methods: Our department performed a study of each patient that we treated for lung cancer using CyberKnife and XLTS. Selection criteria required primary or recurring stage T1 or T2 non–small cell lung cancer and a tumor size of 15-60 mm. Initial staging included a computed tomography scan and 18-F fluorodeoxyglucose positron emission tomography.

Results: We used XLTS to treat fifty-one patients who were not amenable to surgery. The median follow-up was 15 months (range, 5-30 months), median tumor size was 24 mm (range, 15-60 mm), and median total dose was 60 Gy (range, 36-60 Gy) delivered in 3 fractions. The actuarial local control rate was 92% (95% CI; range, 84-99%) at 1 year and 86% (95% CI; range, 75-97%) at 2 years. The actuarial overall survival was 85.5% (95% CI; range, 74.5-96%) at 1 year and 79.4% (95% CI; range, 64-94.8%) at 2 years.

Conclusion: Local control and overall survival rates were similar to those in studies that used fiducials to track tumors. Because XLTS does not require implanted fiducials, patients who were treated with XLTS reported lower toxicity than those who were treated with fiducials. We thus conclude that the fiducial-free method that XLTS makes available to track respiratory motion is a valid option for the most fragile patients.

Introduction

Several methods are currently available which can deliver very high doses of radiation to small volumes of tissue. The precision that is necessary to deliver these doses can be achieved with several techniques, one of which involves tracking the tumor's movement in real time while the patient breathes freely (XLTS). Additionally, patients who have lung cancer and are not amenable to surgery are increasingly being treated with stereotactic body radiation therapy (SBRT). The CyberKnife® Robotic Radiosurgery System (Accuray Incorporated, Sunnyvale, California, USA) was first introduced in France in 2006 through the financial support of the French National Cancer Institute. CyberKnife can deliver SBRT to lung cancer and also simultaneously offer real-time target and motion tracking. It currently features 2 target tracking methods. The first method, fiducial tracking, requires that radiopaque markers be implanted near or inside the tumor, while the second method, the Xsight® Lung Tracking System (XLTS) is fiducial-free. Both tumor tracking methods can be used with the Synchrony® Respiratory Motion Tracking System. This software synchronizes the beams that CyberKnife delivers to the target motion that results from the patient's respiration. While the combined use of Synchrony and fiducial tracking is well documented, the efficacy and toxicity of Synchrony and the fiducial-free tracking of XLTS has not been as thoroughly studied.

Transthoracic fiducial implantation is responsible for the cases of pneumothorax that have been reported in 13% of the patients that undergo this procedure.[1] As some studies have reported pneumothorax rates of 23% or even 38% in transthoracic biopsies[2-5], the rate of 13% may actually be an underestimate. And considering that the concerned population of patients is often very fragile (e.g., elderly patients and/or those with chronic lung disease or other malignancies), the risk of pneumothorax should not be taken lightly. In fact, patients are sometimes excluded from transthoracic fiducial implantation only because they cannot afford the risk of pneumothorax. Fortunately, other fiducial implantation techniques are available, such as electromagnetic navigation-guided bronchoscopy or intravascular coil placement. However, in addition to causing pneumothorax, the radiomarkers that are used in endovascular coils can also cause arrhythmias. In order for the tracking system to work, these radiomarkers must be very precisely inserted, but they occasionally migrate and cause a systematic error at each treatment session. Finally, because results improve when the planning CT is performed a few days after fiducial insertion, the need for fiducials may delay treatment.

With these difficulties in mind, XLTS has been developed to directly track the tumor instead of the fiducials. This new approach may thus represent a shorter and completely nonpresent a shorter, completely uninvasive treatment for patients with lung cancer who are not amenable to surgery.

Our study will address the technical aspects of XLTS, the precise patient selection criteria required for its application, and the efficacy and toxicity outcomes for the 51 patients treated at our center between November 2008 and January 2011. Pulmonary tumors that are > 15 mm and located in the peripheral or apex regions are visible in the orthogonal X-ray images created by the CyberKnife System. These tumors are directly tracked by matching the image intensity pattern of the tumor region in the digitally reconstructed radiographs (DRRs) to the corresponding region in the treatment X-ray images (Figure 1). A correlation model, which will be used during treatment, is then generated by estimating the positions of the internal tumor at different phases of the breathing cycle to the positions of the simultaneous external marker. The alignment of each CyberKnife treatment beam is maintained in real time via the beam's dynamic movement with the target. Phantom experiments that have used XLTS to track tumors report a total system error of 1.07 mm [6-10].

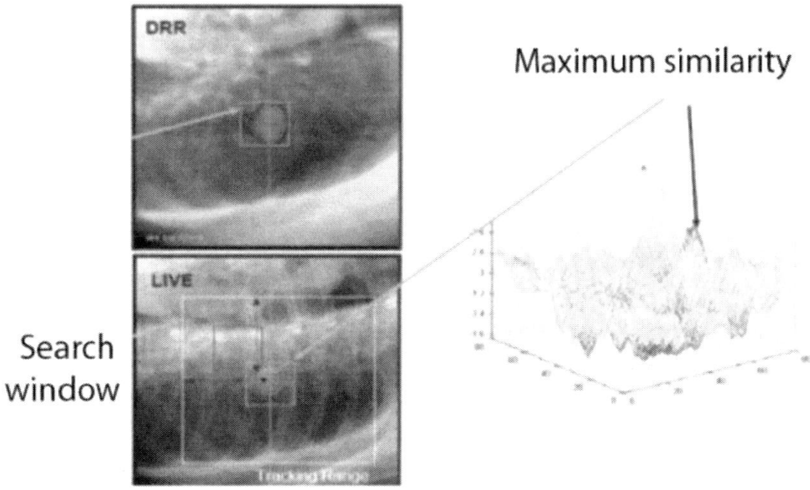

Figure 1. Upper-left corner: treatment planning DRR; Lower-left corner: live imaging from the CyberKnife; Right image: XLTS searching for the optimal similarity between DRR and real-time patient movement.

Patient Eligibility

Patient inclusion criteria for our study required that a single primary or recurring T1 or T2 stage pulmonary lesion with a diameter between 15-60 mm and without lymph node involvement or distant metastases received treatment between November 1, 2008, and January 1, 2011. Initial staging included a computed tomography (CT) scan (thoracic, abdominal, and pelvic) and a 18F-fluorodeoxyglucose–positron emission tomography (FDG-PET) scan. Histological proof was obtained using transthoracic or bronchoscopic biopsy. If histological proof could not be obtained, patients were treated when the lesion was considered "evolutive" (i.e., increasing in size on 2 consecutive CT-scans with an uptake of FDG on a single PET). Any infectious process in the lung, particularly tuberculosis, was investigated and ruled out before the lesion was treated. Other inclusion criteria included an Eastern Cooperative Oncology Group Performance Status of < 2 and no history of an additional neoplasm. Each case was discussed by a radiation oncologist, medical oncologist, radiologist and thoracic surgeon during our thoracic oncology department staff meeting. Lesions were considered surgically removable in patients who were not amenable to surgery. The main reasons for patient inoperability included pre-existing medical conditions such as advanced chronic obstructive pulmonary disease (at the GOLD 3 stage and with a predicted FEV1 of < 49%), cardiovascular disease (with an ejection fraction of < 40%), or general contraindications to anesthesia such as obesity (a BMI of > 30 kg/m2) or a history of anaphylactic shock in response to anesthesia. Although it was acceptable for patients to have previous contralateral or ipsilateral lung surgery or radiation therapy to the treated lesion, our study patients did not receive chemotherapy before, during, or after treatment. Written informed consent was obtained from each patient.

To enable its detection of tumors, XLTS requires that a tumor's diameter be ≥ 15 mm and located inside the lung parenchyma and ≥ 15 mm from any major vascular structure or ribs. The CyberKnife's X-ray tube angulation cannot treat a tumor on the spine that is at a 45° angle.

Treatment Planning, Dose Calculation, and Treatment Session

A thin-sliced CT scan without contrast was recorded with millimetric slices for each patient. The gross tumor volume (GTV) and organs at risk (spinal cord, left and right lungs, heart, and esophagus) were contoured on a CT scan using a window and level setting of -600/1600 HU. A geometrical 3 mm margin was added to the GTV to create the planning target volume (PTV). Treatments were planned using Multiplan® software (Accuray Incorporated, Sunnyvale, California, USA). The dose was calculated using the ray tracing algorithm and prescribed to the 83% isodose line. Dose constraints were as follow: the total lung volume (defined as the right and left lungs, excluding the PTV) that received 5 Gy was < 50% (V5 < 50%; V10 < 30%); for the heart, the maximal dose was < 30 Gy (V24 < 15 $cm^{3)}$; for the trachea and bronchi, the maximum acceptable point doses were 30 Gy (V15 < 4 $cm^{3;}$ V20 < 1 cm^3); for the esophagus, the maximum dose was 25 Gy (V21 < 5 cm^3).

Study Endpoints

Although the XLTS has already been validated on phantom experiments [13-17], its clinical validity has not yet been reported. The primary objective of this study was to evaluate the local control rate that can be achieved with

XLTS. The secondary objective was to evaluate toxicity associated with the use of XLTS. Local control was calculated from the time of treatment until the relapse of the tumor within the PTV. Patients without local relapse were censored on the day of their last follow-up. Local relapse was defined as a 20% increase of the maximum diameter of the tumor on a CT scan as compared to its diameter at initial staging. Overall survival was calculated from the start of radiotherapy until patient death from any cause. Disease-specific survival was measured from the start of radiotherapy until death from lung cancer. Patients that were alive at their last follow-ups were censored. Follow-ups included a CT scan at 3, 6, 9, and 12 months after treatment and every 6 months after that; an FDG-PET was conducted every 6 months. Treatment response was evaluated according to the Response Evaluation Criteria In Solid Tumors v1.1 (RECIST)[11]. Toxicity was evaluated according to the National Cancer Institute's Common Terminology Criteria for Adverse Events (CTCAE) v4.0.

Statistics

SPSS (SPSS Inc., Chicago, Illinois, USA) v13 software was used for statistical analyses. The Kaplan-Meier method with 95% confidence intervals was used to estimate local control and overall and disease-specific survival. Cox regression analysis was used to find the prognostic values of patient and tumor characteristics on local control and overall and disease-specific survival endpoints. Differences between groups were illustrated with Kaplan-Meier curves and the log-rank test. All tests were two-sided. A significance level of $\alpha = 0.05$ was used.

Results

Patient Characteristics

Fifty-one patients were treated with XLTS for non–small cell lung cancer between November 1, 2008, and January 1, 2011. None of these patients were eligible for surgery. Forty-three (84%) of them were men and 8 (16%) were women. The median age was 69 years (range, 50–85 years). All of the patients had been smokers who had quit before XLTS treatment. Histology was known for 19 patients (38%): 10 (20%) had squamous-cell carcinomas, 6 (12%) had adenocarcinomas, and 3 (6%) had undifferentiated cancers. Thirty-one patients had T1 tumors and 20 patients had T2 tumors. The median tumor size was 24 mm (range, 15–60 mm). Eight patients were treated for tumor recurrence after prior surgery (n = 5) or radiation therapy (n = 3). All 51 patients received a FDG-PET scan before treatment with XLTS. Treatment with XLTS obviated the necessity to implant fiducials, thus preventing common sequelae such as pneumothorax. The median delivered dose was 60 Gy (range, 45-60 Gy); a dose of 20 Gy was typically delivered in 3 fractions. However, if the tumor was considered too close to mediastinal structures, the dose/fraction was lowered to 15 Gy and 4 fractions were given; 3 patients received this alternative schedule. The median GTV was 11 cm^3 (range, 1.6-115 cm^3) and the median PTV was 25 cm^3 (range, 4-142 cm^3). The median number of beams used was 70 (range, 20-163 beams) and the median treatment session duration was 63 minutes (range, 27-134 minutes). The dose was prescribed to the 84% isodose line. Median follow-up was 15 months (range, 5-30 months). Actuarial local control was 92% (95% CI = 84-99%) at 1 year and 86% (95% CI = 75-97%) at 2 years (Figure 2). Five patients (10%) experienced local failure in addition to distant metastases to the bone (n = 3), liver (n = 1), brain (n = 2), or contralateral lung (n = 2).

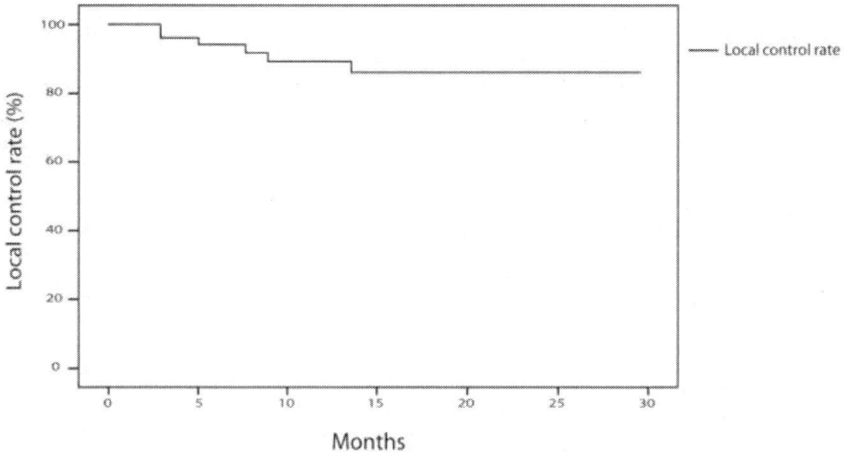

Figure 2. Local control rates of patients treated with the XLTS (n = 51).

Due to radiation pneumonitis that surrounded the treated tumor, 1 patient's response to the treatment could not be evaluated on the first CT scan at 3 months. However, that patient's evaluation at 12 months showed a complete resolution of the pneumonitis and a partial response. One patient relapsed with mediastinal lymph node metastases 2 years after treatment.

Actuarial overall survival was 85.5% (95% CI; range, 74.5-96%) at 1 year and 79.4% (95% CI; range, 64-94.8%) at 2 years. Seven patients died during follow-up, 5 from cancer progression and 2 from intercurrent disease. Actuarial disease-specific survival was 90.1% (95% CI; range, 71-100%) at 1 year and 84% (95% CI; range, 69-98%) at 2 years.

Prognostic Factors for Overall Survival and Local Control

Patient, tumor, and treatment characteristics were investigated as prognostic factors for overall survival and local control. With regard to overall survival, no significant difference was found based on sex ($p = 0.254$), age ($p = 0.512$), availability of histologic data ($p = 0.190$), total dose delivered ($p = 0.705$), or number of fractions ($p = 0.543$). However, patients with a maximum tumor diameter of < 3 cm tended to have better overall survival ($p = 0.052$). A GTV of > 10 cm^3 was significantly associated with poorer survival (100% vs. 65.2% at 2 years, $p = 0.029$; see Figure 3).

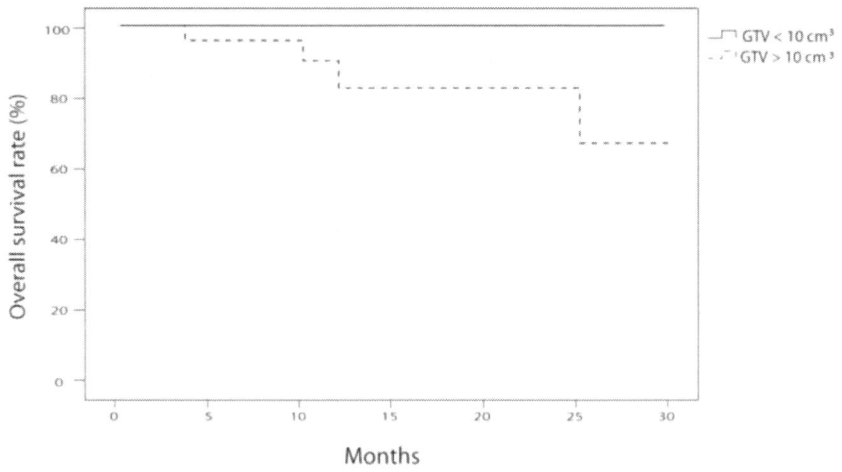

Figure 3. Overall survival of patients with a GTV > 10 cm^3 (n = 23) and patients with GTV < 10 cm^3 (n = 28) treated with the XLTS ($p = 0.029$).

Regarding local control, no significant difference was observed based on sex ($p = 0.886$), age ($p = 0.26$), availability of histologic data ($p = 0.98$), tumor size (p = 0.224), GTV (p = 0.171), or total dose delivered (p = 0.33). However, a significant difference was found between patients who were treated with 3 fractions and patients who were treated with > 3 fractions. Specifically, the local control rate at 2 years was 100% for patients treated with 3 fractions, but 70% for patients treated with > 3 fractions (p = 0.006; see Figure 4).

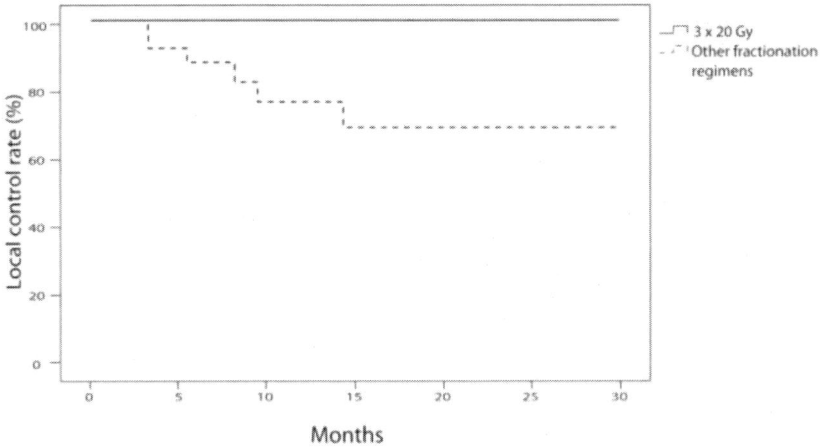

Figure 4. The local control rates of patients who were treated with 3 fractions (n = 27) and patients who were treated with > 3 fractions (n = 24) of XLTS (p = 0.006).

Toxicity

Because XLTS does not require fiducials for tumor tracking, no cases of pneumothorax were observed. Seven cases (14%) of grade 1 radiation pneumonitis without any clinical impact and 1 grade 2 (2%) radiation pneumonitis were observed at 3 months. None of these patients required steroids. Three grade 1 (6%) radiation fibroses were observed on a CT scan that was performed 1 year after treatment. No acute or late grade 3 or 4 toxicities were observed.

Discussion

Several studies discussing SBRT for early-stage lung cancer have been published. After White et al., published a dose-escalation study in 2003, series reporting of patients treated with CyberKnife began to emerge. In 2006, Nuyttens et al., wrote about 20 patients that were treated for 22 lung tumors [12]. These researchers chose a treatment that required the use of 78 markers to track the tumors: 34 were implanted using transthoracic punction, 23 were endovascular coils, and 21 were extrathoracic. No cases of pneumothorax were reported. The local control rate was 100% at 4 months. In 2007, Collins et al., published a study of 25 patients who were also treated using fiducials [13]. Seven of the 25 patients presented with pneumothorax. Another study published in 2008 by Castelli et al., involved close to 30 patients and reported 4 cases of pneumothorax and 1 fiducial migration [14]. The study with the most patients was published in 2009 by van der Voort van Zyp et al. [15] Seventy surgery-ineligible patients (39 with T1 tumors and 31 with T2 tumors) were treated with 45 Gy or 60 Gy in 3 fractions. The local control rate was 96% for the patients who were treated with 60 Gy and 78% for the patients who were treated with 45 Gy. A total of 225 fiducials were used (143 endovascular coils, 72 implanted using bronchoscopy, and 10 implanted by transthoracic punction). Tumor tracking for each patient required 1-5 fiducials. This fiducial implantation induced 2 grade 3 toxicities (1 pneumothorax requiring a chest drain and 1 arrhythmia following intravascular coil placement), 1 grade 2 toxicity (pneumothorax), and 6 grade 1 toxicities (dyspnea, n = 1; pneumothorax, n = 2; self-limiting haemorrhage, n = 3). Although toxicities were not frequent, they should not be overlooked.

Our study is the first, to our knowledge, to report only on patients who were treated with a fiducial-free method of tumor tracking. We reported a local control rate of 88% at 15 months, which is comparable to other studies and indicates that XLTS can be used without a loss in efficacy. However, a treatment time of > 60 minutes can potentially lead to a biological equivalent dose (BED) loss to the tumor of > 10-15%, a loss which significantly impacts tumor control[15]. The median treatment time for our patients was 63 minutes (range, 27-134 minutes) and may explain our local failure rate. In order to decrease the time spent in CyberKnife treatments, the number of pencil beams should therefore be kept to a minimum.

Patients treated with ≥ 4 fractions had worse local control rate than patients treated with 3 fractions. This difference can be explained by the fact that a lower BED resulted when an increased number of sessions with the same total dose was delivered (i.e., the BED for 60 Gy/4 fractions was 150 Gy while the BED for 60 Gy/3 fractions was 180 Gy). The number of treatment sessions should thus be kept to 3.

Five patients (10%) with local control relapsed with distant metastases to the bone (n = 3), liver (n = 1), brain (n = 2), or the contralateral lung (n = 2). One patient relapsed with mediastinal lymph node metastases 2 years after treatment. A major limitation of our study was the small number of patients with known histology (38%), a common scenario in SBRT studies for lung cancer. Van der Voort van Zyp et al., reported an absence of confirmation of malignancy in 49% of their study patients. Also worth noting is the fact that most patients receive SBRT treatment because they are too fragile for surgery or even transthoracic biopsies. Swensen et al., created a malignancy prediction model that, combined with FDG-PET [16], could be useful in calculating unknown histologies.

We reported 7 grade 1 (14%) and 2 grade 2 (14%) cases of radiation pneumonitis and no grade 3 or 4 incidents. These rates are lower than those that have been reported in other studies (i.e., grade 3 toxicities of 3-10%) [17-19]. The fact that none of our patients had any post-treatment pain or rib fractures may be due to our study's strict selection criteria (which mandated that all treated tumors be ≥ 15 mm from the ribs). We observed 3 cases of grade 1 lung fibrosis.

There is an important need for multicenter randomized trials that will compare surgery to SBRT. To address this need, an international randomized prospective trial (STARS, ClinicalTrials.gov ID: NCT00840749) was initiated by Accuray in collaboration with the MD Anderson Cancer Center (Texas, USA) in December 2008 to compare surgery to SBRT for operable patients with early-stage non–small cell lung cancer tumors < 4 cm in diameter and without lymph node or distant metastases. Surgeries that are included in this trial include lobectomy, bilobectomy, or pneumonectomy. The primary endpoint is overall survival. Meanwhile, the European multicenter randomized trial (ROSEL, ClinicalTrials.gov ID: NCT00687986) that compared SBRT to surgery for operable patients has recently been terminated due to poor recruitment.

Conclusion

SBRT to the lung using fiducial-free tumor tracking (XLTS) is both feasible and effective. The local control rate is similar to what other studies found when markers were implanted to track tumors. Additionally, the delivery of treatment without the use of fiducials led to a lower toxicity which prevented the cases of pneumothorax that are normally associated with this procedure. However, precise patient selection according to simple criteria was required for the XLTS to work. This System is an intriguing treatment option for patients who are not amenable to surgery or are too fragile for transthoracic punction and fiducial implantation. A standard 3 x 20-Gy fractionation regimen should be used to achieve optimal local control.

SBRT is increasingly being used to treat early-stage lung cancer. Methods that are available to achieve its necessary precision include respiratory gating, a body frame, or real-time tumor tracking. Real-time tumor tracking can be performed with fiducials or with the new method (XLTS) that tracks the tumor itself. We reported the first clinical study using this fiducial-free treatment. With local control rates of 92% and 86% at 1 and 2 years, respectively, the results of this method seem comparable to other studies that use fiducials.

References

[1] Whyte RI, Crownover R, Murphy MJ. et al. Stereotactic radiosurgery for lung tumors: preliminary report of a phase I trial. *Ann Thor Surg*. 2003;75:1097. doi: 10.1016/S0003-4975(02)04681-7. [PubMed] [Cross Ref]

[2] Geraghty PR, Kee ST, McFarlane G. et al. CT-guided Transthoracic Needle Aspiration Biopsy of Pulmonary Nodules: Needle Size and Pneumothorax Rate. *Radiology*. 2003;229:475–481. doi: 10.1148/radiol.2291020499. [PubMed] [Cross Ref]

[3] Saji H, Nakamura H, Tsuchida T. et al. The Incidence and the Risk of Pneumothorax and Chest Tube Placement After Percutaneous CT-Guided Lung Biopsy. *Chest*. 2002;121:1521–1526. doi: 10.1378/chest.121.5.1521. [PubMed] [Cross Ref]

[4] Reichner CA, Collins BT, Gagnon GJ. et al. The placement of gold fiducials for CyberKnife stereotactic radiosurgery using a modified transbronchial needle aspiration technique. *J Bronchol*. 2005;12:193. doi: 10.1097/01.lab.0000186345.85025.41. [Cross Ref]

[5] Yeow KM, Su I. et al. Risk Factors of Pneumothorax and Bleeding. *Chest*. 2004;126:748. doi: 10.1378/chest.126.3.748. [PubMed] [Cross Ref]

[6] Fu D, Kahn R, Wang B. et al. Fiducial-free Lung Tumor Tracking for CyberKnife Radiosurgery. *Int J Radiat Oncol Biol Phys*. 2008;72:S608–S609.

[7] Fu D, Kuduvalli G. Enhancing skeletal features in digitally reconstructed radiographs. *Image Processing*.Vol 6144, San Diego, CA, USA; 2006.

[8] Sayeh S, Wang J, Main W, Kilby W, Maurer C. Respiratory Motion Tracking for Robotic Radiosurgery. D*ans: Treating Tumors that Move with Respiration. Springer*. Urschel, Harold C. 2007;15:15–29.

[9] Schweikard A, Glosser G, Bodduluri M, Murphy MJ, Adler JR. Robotic motion compensation for respiratory movement during radiosurgery. *Comput Aided Surg*. 2000;5:263–277. doi: 10.3109/1092908 0009148894. [PubMed] [Cross Ref]

[10] Schweikard A, Shiomi H, Adler J. Respiration tracking in radiosurgery. *Med Phys*. 2004;31:2738. doi: 10.1118/1.1774132. [PubMed] [Cross Ref]

[11] Therasse P, Arbuck SG, Eisenhauer EA. et al. New guidelines to evaluate the response to treatment in solid tumors. European Organization for Research and Treatment of Cancer, National Cancer Institute of the United States, National Cancer Institute of Canada. J. 2000;92:205–216. doi: 10.1093/jnci/92.3.205. [PubMed] [Cross Ref]

[12] Nuyttens JJ, Prévost J-B, Praag J. et al. Lung tumor tracking during stereotactic radiotherapy treatment with the CyberKnife: Marker placement and early results. *Acta Oncol.* 2006;45:961–965. doi: 10.1080/02841860600902205. [PubMed] [Cross Ref]

[13] Collins B, Erickson K, Reichner C. et al. Radical stereotactic radiosurgery with real-time tumor motion tracking in the treatment of small peripheral lung tumors. *Radiat Oncol*. 2007;2:39. doi: 10.1186/1748-717X-2-39. [PMC free article] [PubMed] [Cross Ref]

[14] Castelli J, Thariat J, Benezery K. et al. Analyse de la toxicité précoce des traitements par Cyberknife® des cancers pulmonaires et résultats préliminaires. *Cancer Radiother*. 2008;12:793–799. doi: 10.1016/j.canrad.2008.06.002. [PubMed] [Cross Ref]

[15] van Zyp NC Van der Voort, Prévost JB, Hoogeman MS. et al. Stereotactic radiotherapy with real-time tumor tracking for non-small cell lung cancer*: Clinical outcome. Radiother Oncol*. 2009;91:296–300. doi: 10.1016/j.radonc.2009.02.011. [PubMed] [Cross Ref]

[16] Herder GJ, Van Tinteren H, Colding RP. et al. Clinical prediction model to characterize pulmonary nodules: Validation and added value of 18 F-fluorodeoxyglucose positron emission tomography. *Chest.* 2005;128:2490–2496. doi: 10.1378/chest.128.4.2490. [PubMed] [Cross Ref]

[17] Aoki T, Nagata Y, Negoro Y. et al. Evaluation of Lung Injury after Three-dimensional Conformal Stereotactic Radiation Therapy for Solitary Lung Tumors: CT Appearance. *Radiology.* 2004;230:101–108. doi: 10.1148/radiol.2301021226. [PubMed] [Cross Ref]

[18] Mehta V. Radiation pneumonitis and pulmonary fibrosis in non–small-cell lung cancer: Pulmonary function, prediction, and prevention. *Int J Radiat Oncol Biol Phys.* 2005;63:5–24. doi: 10.1016j.ijrobp. 2005.03.047. [PubMed] [Cross Ref]

[19] Takeda T, Takeda A, Kunieda E. et al. Radiation injury after hypofractionated stereotactic radiotherapy for peripheral small lung tumors: serial changes on CT. *Am J Roentgenol.* 2004;182:1123. [PubMed]

Part III: CyberKnife Treatment

In: The Revolution of Robotic …
Editor: Pierre-Yves Bondiau
ISBN: 978-1-62808-718-5

Chapter 10

CyberKnife with Fiducial Tracking for Inoperable Peripheral Stage I Non-Small Cell Lung Cancer (NSCLC): Locoregional Control and Overall Survival Outcomes

Brian T. Collins[*], *Eric K. Oermann*, *Shaan Kataria*, *Catherine Jamis*, *Saloomeh Vahdat*, *Leonard Chen*, *Simeng Suy*, *Sean P. Collins* *and Eric Anderson*
Georgetown University Hospital, Washington, DC. US

Abstract

Associated comorbidities or advanced age prevent many patients with clinical stage I non-small cell lung carcinoma (NSCLC) from undergoing surgery. For patients such as these, the CyberKnife and its use of fiducial tracking may provide the optimal treatment. In this chapter

[*] Email: collinsb@gunet.georgetown.edu.

we will provide a brief overview of Georgetown University Hospital's current treatment approach using the CyberKnife. We will also review its mature outcomes for inoperable stage I NSCLC patients that were treated with the CyberKnife and fiducial tracking.

Introduction

Georgetown University Hospital was among the first institutions in the world to employ the CyberKnife system. Following the 2003 [1] publication of early and favorable stage I NSCLC outcomes using stereotactic body radiation therapy (SBRT), Georgetown University Hospital purchased the CyberKnife Synchrony motion tracking module and implemented a treatment policy for eligible patients. Patients that were to be included in this review were evaluated by the Georgetown University Hospital multidisciplinary thoracic oncology team, which consisted of staff thoracic surgeons, pulmonologists, pathologists, medical oncologists, radiologists, and radiation oncologists. Per institutional policy, all patients required pathologic confirmation of malignancy prior to treatment and completed pretreatment PET/CT imaging and pulmonary function testing.

Patients and Method

Prior to proceeding with treatment planning, 3-5 gold fiducial markers measuring 1 mm in diameter by 5 mm in length were placed in close proximity to the tumors under CT guidance for tumor motion tracking. Although this method has a known risk of pneumothorax, it was initially chosen in order to optimize the positioning and spacing of the fiducials. Currently, however, it is our institutional preference to place fiducials via bronchoscopy. [2,3] This latter approach has not resulted (to date) in pneumothoraces, but instead allows for mediastinal lymph node staging and visual confirmation of the integrity of major airways prior to treatment. [4]

Following fiducial placement, fine-cut (1.25 mm) treatment planning CT scans were obtained during a full inhalation breath hold in the supine treatment position. Lung windows were used to contour gross tumor volumes (GTV) and a treatment plan using a 5-mm margin was generated. After passing through collimators with 20-35 mm diameters, hundreds of small beams were then spread out over a large solid angle that optimized the dose distribution for each patient and resulted in a relatively high dose to the central tumor and dose gradients that closely conformed to the shape of the target. This treatment approach is the theoretical ideal for treating the radiation-resistant tumor center and the spread of radiation-sensitive subclinical radial disease that is seen with NSCLC. The radiation dose was prescribed to an isodose line that covered at least 95% of the planning treatment volume (GTV + 5 mm). All critical thoracic structures were contoured in order to ensure that the incidental radiation on these structures was tracked and limited. The percentage of the total lung volume receiving more than 15 Gy was also tracked and limited to 15%. Radiation was delivered in 3 or 5 fractions of 10-20 Gy each for a total dose of 45-60 Gy to the prescription isodose line (Biologic Equivalent Dose (BED) $Gy_{10} > 100$ Gy). Fractions were 1-2 hours long and delivered over 3-11 days. Lower doses or additional fractions were prescribed when concerns about adjacent structures arose or when patients had very severe cardiopulmonary dysfunction.

When considering patients for this analysis it was necessary to confirm that their tumors were, in fact, peripheral. However, at the onset of this research, "peripheral" lesions in SBRT had only recently been conservatively defined by the Radiation Therapy Oncology Group as those that lay at least 2 cm from the major central airways (i.e., carina, main bronchi, upper lobe bronchi, intermedius bronchus, middle lobe bronchus, lingular bronchus, and lower lobe bronchi). We chose to more inclusively define peripheral lesions as tumors that were located far enough away from sensitive central structures so that high doses of radiation (10-20 Gy/fraction) could be delivered to them while still adhering to published dose limits for adjacent critical structures. [5] Our use of this novel definition has allowed for the vast majority of inoperable stage I NSCLC patients that are evaluated at Georgetown University Hospital to become candidates for the described CyberKnife treatment approach. Furthermore, using this definition, we have not found severe toxicity in stage I NSCLC patients.

In preparation for treatment delivery, patients were placed unrestrained on the treatment couch in the supine position with their arms at their sides and allowed to breathe freely. Patient positioning was optimized through the use of the digitally reconstructed radiographic images that were derived from the planning CT images. Patients wore a form-fitting vest and 3 red LEDs were placed on its anterior surface in the region of maximum chest and upper abdominal excursion. These LEDs were visible to an adjustable camera array in the treatment room.

Table 1. Patient and tumor characteristics

FEV1 (L)	
Median	0.99
Range	0.53-3.06
% predicted FEV1	
Median	61
Range	21-108
DLCO (mL/min/mmHg)	
Median	9.3
Range	5.1-23.3
% predicted DLCO	
Median	52
Range	33-128
ECOG score	
Median	1
Range	0-3
Age (years)	
Median	76
Range	62-94
Sex (%)	
Male	30
Female	70
Race (%)	
Caucasian	73
African-American	27
Smoker (%)	95
Histology (%)	
Adenocarcinoma	47.5
Squamous-cell cancer	32.5
NSCLC NOS	20.0
Clinical stage (%)	
T1 N0	67.5
T2 N0	32.5
Maximum diameter (cm)	
Median	2.7
Range	1.4-5.0

FEV1: forced expiratory volume in 1 second.
DLCO: carbon monoxide diffusing capacity.
ECOG: Eastern Cooperative Oncology Group.
NOS: not otherwise specified.

The location of the fiducials could be seen in the multiple orthogonal x-ray images that were acquired by ceiling-mounted diagnostic x-ray sources and corresponding floor-mounted amorphous-silicon image detectors located on both sides of the patient.

Prior to initiating treatment, an adaptive correlation model was produced between the positions of the fiducials (as periodically imaged by the x-ray targeting system) and the red light-emitting markers (as continuously imaged by the camera array). A valid model requires a minimum of 3 x-ray images and, optimally, the last 10 fiducial images that were taken at varying points in the respiratory cycle. To verify treatment and update the correlation model, the fiducials were imaged prior to the delivery of every third beam during treatment. If the fiducials were misidentified by the software or the correlation error exceeded 3 mm in more than 1 consecutive image, the treatment was stopped and the model was rebuilt with 3 images and optimized with additional images. The marker signal and correlation model tracked the tumor's position during treatment. To maintain alignment with the tumor throughout the complete respiratory cycle, the computer-controlled robotic arm moved the lightweight 6-MV X-band LINAC while hundreds of radiation beams were delivered to the target.

Clinical examination and PET/CT imaging were performed at follow-up intervals of 3-6 months. Locoregional recurrence was defined as NSCLC progression in the involved lobe or regional lymph nodes (per the serial PET/CT imaging that was previously described [6]). Other failures were considered distant and biopsy was required to confirm disease progression.

Results

Forty patients (12 men and 28 women) with clinical stage I NSCLC (19 with adenocarcinoma, 13 with squamous-cell carcinoma, and 8 with not-otherwise-specified NSCLC) were treated over a 72-month period between August 2005 and August 2011 (Table 1). Ninety-five percent of these patients were smokers; pulmonary dysfunction was the primary rationale for nonsurgical treatment for 60% of all patients. The median percent of predicted forced expiratory volume in 1 second was 61% (range, 21-108%). The remaining patients (40%) were at least 75 years old and did not wish to pursue surgery. The median maximum tumor diameter was 2.7 cm (range, 1.4-5.0 cm). Patients who were excluded from this analysis included those who had a history of pneumonectomy, thoracic irradiation, and/or malignancy in the last

5 years and/or were treated with palliative intent (BED $Gy_{10} < 100$ Gy) were excluded from this analysis.

Table 2. Treatment characteristics

	Median (Range)
Prescribed dose (Gy)	50 (45-60)
Prescription isodose line (%)	80 (75-85)
Number of fractions	3 (3-5)
Number of beams per treatment	176 (119-266)
Treatment course (days)	7 (3-13)
% of total lung volume receiving at least 15 Gy	6.2 (2.4-12.9)

Treatment plans were composed of a median 176 pencil beams (Table 2). A median dose of 50 Gy was delivered to the prescription isodose line in 3 or 5 treatments of 1-2 hours each over a 3-13 day period (median, 7 days). The total lung volume that received at least 15 Gy was 6.2% (range, 2.4-12.9%). None of the patients received adjuvant chemotherapy or therapeutic mediastinal radiation therapy.

All patients who had persistent tumor maximum standardized uptake value elevations following treatment were biopsied. Two local and 5 distant failures were pathologically confirmed during follow-up. At a median follow-up of 33 months (range, 20-92 months), the 3- and 5-year Kaplan-Meier locoregional controls were both 94% (Figure 1), and the 3- and 5-year overall survival estimates were 71% and 34%, respectively (Figure 2). Twelve of the 18 deaths were attributed to cardiopulmonary dysfunction.

The 2 patients with pathologically confirmed local failure developed metastases that resulted in their deaths 3 years following CyberKnife treatment. Five patients with controlled primaries developed metastases that led to 3 of their deaths (to date).

Three patients developed second primaries (2 lung and 1 bile duct); one died of second primary metastatic disease, one died of pulmonary dysfunction, and the third, an 80-year-old patient with a second bile duct primary, is alive and without evidence of disease following surgery and adjuvant chemotherapy. Four patients have been alive for at least 5 years and are also without evidence of disease.

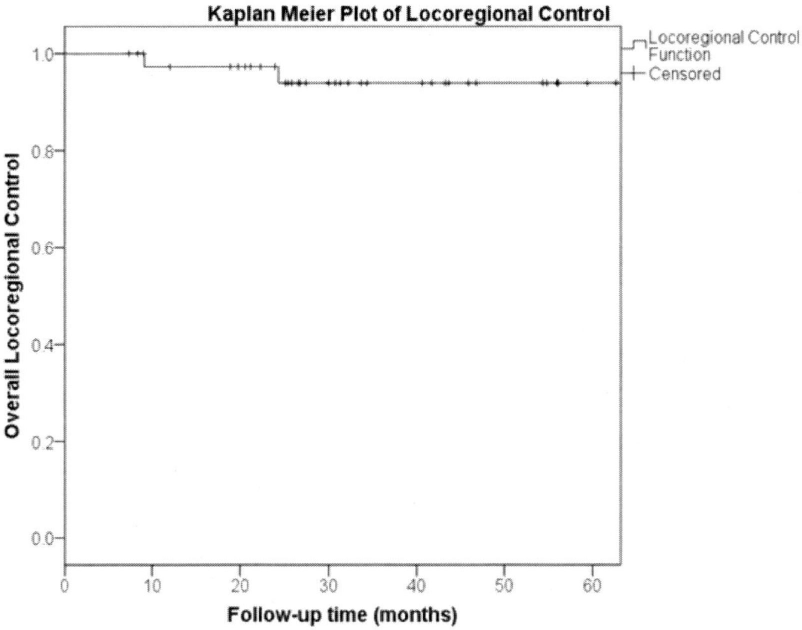

Figure 1. Kaplan-Meier plot of locoregional control.

Discussion

Based on the early and promising SBRT findings published in late 2003 [1], we began using CyberKnife to treat patients with inoperable peripheral stage I NSCLC. Because the fiducials allowed us to continuously track tumor motion during treatment, we were able to deliver conformal dose distributions with tight margins (5 mm) around the tumors. Hundreds of beams were used to produce a relatively high dose to the central tumor and steep uniform dose gradients that conformed closely to the shape of the tumors. We limited the maximum point doses that were delivered to critical normal structures and used these limits to help define lesions as "peripheral"; the vast majority of stage I patients treated at Georgetown University Hospital are now considered to have peripheral NSCLC and are thus eligible for radical CyberKnife treatment. Forty patients were treated in 6 years and followed for a minimum of 20 months. At a median follow-up of 33 months, the 3- and 5-year Kaplan-Meier locoregional controls were both 94% and the 3- and 5-year overall survival estimates were 71% and 34%, respectively. Four patients are alive and have been disease-free for at least 5 years; they are thus considered cured.

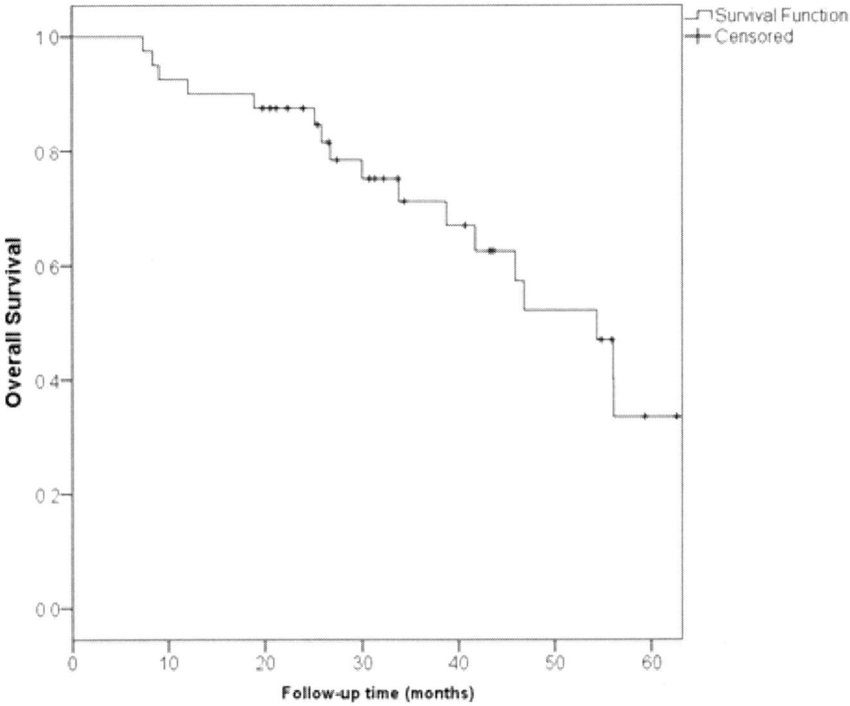

Figure 2. Kaplan-Meier plot of overall survival.

Conclusion

CyberKnife with fiducial tracking is a curative treatment option for clinical stage I NSCLC. The need to reliably treat small moving targets with tight margins throughout the thoracic cavity requires such an optimal radiation delivery system with robust image verification. Impressive late locoregional control rates (94%) and the existence of long-term and disease-free survivors has prompted us to use CyberKnife to treat high-risk but operable patients whose only surgical treatment option is wedge resection. [7]

References

[1] Timmerman R, Papiez L, McGarry R, *et al.* Extracranial stereotactic radioablation: results of a phase I study in medically inoperable stage I non-small cell lung cancer. *Chest* 2003;124:1946-1955.

[2] Reichner CA, Collins BT, Gagnon GJ, *et al.* The placement of gold fiducials for CyberKnife stereotactic radiosurgery using a modified transbronchial needle aspiration technique. *Journal of Bronchology* 2005;12:193-195.

[3] Harley DP, Krimsky WS, Sarkar S, et al. Fiducial marker placement using endobronchial ultrasound and navigational bronchoscopy for stereotactic radiosurgery: an alternative strategy. *Ann Thorac Surg.* 2010;89(2):368-73.

[4] Sarwate D, Sarkar S, Krimsky WS, et al. Optimization of mediastinal staging in potential candidates for stereotactic radiosurgery of the chest. *J Thorac Cardiovasc Surg.* 2012;144(1):81-6.

[5] Benedict SH, Yenice KM, Followill D, et al. Stereotactic body radiation therapy; the report of AAPM Task Group 101. *Med Phys.* 2010;37(8):4078-101.

[6] Vahdat, S., Oermann, E.K., Collins, S.P., et al. CyberKnife radiosurgery for inoperable stage IA non-small cell lung cancer: 18F-fluorodeoxyglucose positron emission tomography/computed tomography serial tumor response assessment. *J Hematol Onco. 2010; l* 3, 6.

[7] Chen VJ, Oermann E, Vahdat S, et al. CyberKnife with Tumor Tracking: An Effective Treatment for High-Risk Surgical Patients with Stage I Non-Small Cell Lung Cancer. *Front Oncol.* 2012;2:9.

In: The Revolution of Robotic …
Editor: Pierre-Yves Bondiau

ISBN: 978-1-62808-718-5

Chapter 11

Central Lung Tumors

Joost Jan Nuyttens *

Department of Radiation Oncology,
Erasmus MC-Daniel den Hoed Cancer Center,
Rotterdam, the Netherlands

Abstract

The CyberKnife is a frameless image-guided radiotherapy system involving a 6-MV linear accelerator mounted on a robotic arm. The imaging system consists of two diagnostic x-ray sources mounted to the ceiling paired with amorphous silicon detectors to acquire live digital radiographic images of the tumor or tumor surrogates including bony anatomy or implanted fiducial markers. We present a review to evaluate local control, overall survival, and toxicity of stereotactic body radiotherapy (SBRT)

Conclusion: SBRT of central lung lesions can be safely delivered, with promising early tumor control in patients many of whom have severe comorbid conditions.

* Corresponding author: Email : j.nuyttens@erasmusmc.nl.

Introduction

The tumor-ablative effects of high-dose stereotactic body radiation therapy (SBRT) for lung cancer can be safely extended to lesions in the central chest if treatment is adapted to reduce the risk of injury to organs at risk (OAR). Several studies have now shown that delivering lower doses of SBRT over 4-10 fractions can reduce toxicity in the central chest [5-11]. However, the doses that are often used to treat peripheral lung lesions can result in serious toxicity and death when delivered to central lesions [1, 2, 4, 12], or at least cause a higher rate of toxicity than for peripheral lesions [3]. As SBRT studies have been infrequent, this chapter will also discuss other findings.

Clinical Outcomes

Published SBRT studies have typically consisted of a mix of peripheral and central tumors and a relatively small number of patients (8-27 patients) with central tumors (Cf. Figure 1). However, 2 studies have reported on larger groups. Haasbeek et al. [4] reported on 63 patients who were treated with 8 fractions of 7.5 Gy. Of these 63 patients, 37 had a tumor at a central hilar location and 26 had tumors abutting the pericardium or mediastinal structures. The median follow-up was 35 months. The 3-year local control (LC) rate was 92.6%, and the 3-year overall survival rate was 64.3%. Late grade III toxicity was limited to chest wall pain (n = 2) and increased dyspnea (n = 2). No grade IV/V toxicity was observed, but grade V toxicity could not be excluded with certainty in 9 patients who died of cardiopulmonary causes.

Nuyttens et al. [16] reported on 58 central lesions in 56 patients (39 with primary, 17 with metastatic tumours). Fifteen tumors located near the esophagus were treated with 6 fractions of 8 Gy. The 43 other tumors were treated according to the following dose escalation scheme: 5 fractions of 9 Gy (n = 6), 5 fractions of 10 Gy (n = 15), and 5 fractions of 12 Gy (n = 22). To protect adjacent OAR, the coverage of the planned target volume was reduced below 95% in 21 patients. At a median follow-up of 23 months, the actuarial 2-year LC was 85% for tumors treated with a biological equivalent dose (BED) > 100 Gy compared to 60% for tumors treated with a BED ≤ 100 Gy.

Some studies that delivered lower fraction doses reported that reduced toxicity seemed to come at the expense of poorer LC. For example, Taremi et al. delivered 50 Gy or 60 Gy in 8 fractions to 20 patients with central lesions (out of a total of 108 treated patients), and observed no severe toxicity related to tumor location [10]. However, 7 of the 10 local recurrences developed in patients with central lesions, 5 of which were treated with 50 Gy.

Chang et al. observed low toxicity but a high recurrence rate (43%) in 7 patients treated to 40 Gy in 4 fractions [8]. A similar combination of low dose (BED < 100 Gy) and relatively low toxicity and LC were obtained by Onimaru et al. [6] and Guckenberger et al. [13]. We treated several of our patients with doses of < 50 Gy, and also found a statistical trend toward poorer LC in these patients, a finding that is consistent with the previously mentioned reports.

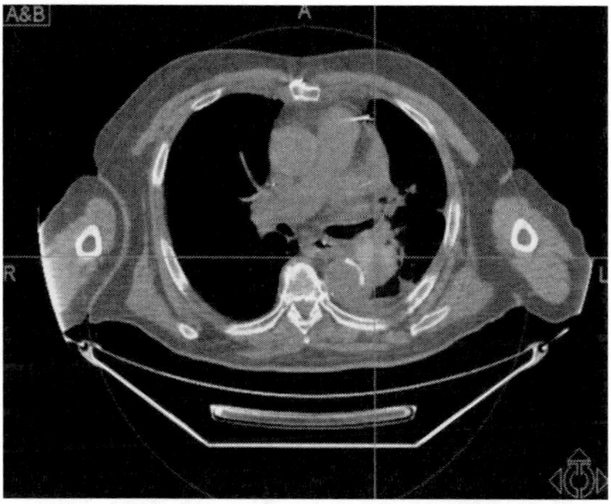

Figure 1. Central tumour according to definition.

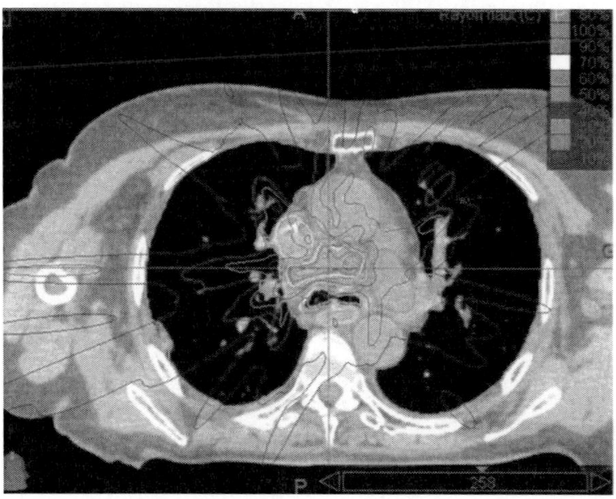

Figure 2. Example of central tumor dosimetry (75Gy/5fr), Avoiding; aorta, carena, esophagus and vena cava (see Annex C for organ at risk constraint).

Other authors, however, have reported the ability to deliver doses ≥ BED 100 Gy and still achieve good tumor control (> 85% at 1.5-2 years) and low toxicity [9, 10, 12]. For example, Stephans et al. were able to treat central lung lesions without serious toxicity using 50 Gy delivered in 5 fractions. Patients were immobilized in a stereotactic frame and abdominal compression was applied to reduce tumor motion. Tumor control at a median follow-up of 18.4 months was 98%.

Some authors have reported low toxicity [9, 10, 12] with the use of relatively high doses of SBRT. However, 5 other publications reported death due to pulmonal complications and 2 due to esophageal complications. Two authors [4, 13] reported the death of 1 patient secondary to bronchial stenosis and subsequent bleeding from the bronchus. In 1 patient, the dose to the tumor was 48 Gy in 4 fractions; in the other patient the dose was not specified (but it was probably 60 Gy in 4 fractions, based on other details in the report). Milano et al. reported 1 death due to fatal hemoptysis after treatment of a mediastinal mass abutting the bronchus [15]; the cumulative dose to the bronchus was 98 Gy. Le et al. reported 2 deaths due to pulmonary complications [1]; both patients had received radiotherapy to the chest. Fakaris et al. reported 5 grade 5 toxicities, all possibly related to the SBRT treatment of 22 patients. Three of these patients died due to pneumonia, one to hemoptysis and one to respiratory failure [5]. Le et al., reported the death of one patient due to esophageal fistula followed by a fatal hemoptysis from a tracheovascular fistula [1].

Brachial plexopathy has been reported in 2 patients: One of these patients developed a brachial plexopathy that was managed medically; however, the dose to the plexus was not reported [7]. The other patient developed brachial plexus neuropathy and partial arm paralysis after receiving a dose of 40 Gy (in 4 fractions) to a significant volume of the plexus [8].

Nuyttens et al. [16] reported on 58 central lesions in 56 patients and did not find any grade 4 or 5 toxicity. He calculated the volume of the OAR that received a certain dose. The median volume of the main bronchi irradiated to a delivered dose in equivalent 2 Gy fractions (EQD2) of 130 Gy or a BED of 216 Gy in 29 patients was 0.4 cm^3 (range, 0.001-4.9 cm^3). The median maximum dose to the esophagus was 88 Gy_3 EQD2 of 143 Gy BED. Acute grade 1-2 esophagitis was observed in 11% of patients.

Conclusion

A risk-adapted treatment of central lesions requires both a consideration of the maximum overall and individual fraction dose. Because several authors reported grade 4 and 5 toxicities, it is also necessary to optimize the dose distribution to meet strict dose constraints for sensitive central structures. The fact that doses as low as 40 Gy can cause significant complications points to the critical importance of careful treatment planning, accurate patient setup, and precise radiation delivery throughout a treatment fraction [13].

References

[1] Le, QT; Loo, BW; Ho, A; et al. Results of a phase I dose-escalation study using single-fraction stereotactic radiotherapy for lung tumors. *J Thorac Oncol*, 2006, 1, 802-809.

[2] Timmerman, R; McGarry, R; Yiannoutsos, C; et al. Excessive toxicity when treating central tumors in a phase II study of stereotactic body radiation therapy for medically inoperable early-stage lung cancer. *J Clin Oncol*, 2006, 24, 4833-4839.

[3] Bral, S; Gevaert, T; Linthout, N; et al. Prospective, Risk-Adapted Strategy of Stereotactic Body Radiotherapy for Early-Stage Non-Small-Cell Lung Cancer: Results of a Phase II Trial. *Int J Radiat Oncol Biol Phys*, 2010.

[4] Haasbeek, CJ; Lagerwaard, FJ; Slotman, BJ; Senan, S. Outcomes of stereotactic ablative radiotherapy for centrally located early-stage lung cancer. *J Thorac Oncol*, 2011 Dec, 6(12), 2036-43.

[5] Fakiris, AJ; McGarry, RC; Yiannoutsos, CT; et al. Stereotactic body radiation therapy for early-stage non-small-cell lung carcinoma: four-year results of a prospective phase II study. *Int J Radiat Oncol Biol Phys*, 2009, 75, 677-682.

[6] Onimaru, R; Shirato, H; Shimizu, S; et al. Tolerance of organs at risk in small-volume, hypofractionated, image-guided radiotherapy for primary and metastatic lung cancers. *Int J Radiat Oncol Biol Phys*, 2003, 56, 126-135.

[7] Bradley, JD; El Naqa, I; Drzymala, RE; Trovo, M; Jones, G; Denning, MD. Stereotactic body radiation therapy for early-stage non-small-cell

lung cancer: the pattern of failure is distant. *Int J Radiat Oncol Biol Phys*, 2010, 77, 1146-1150.

[8] Chang, JY; Balter, PA; Dong, L; et al. Stereotactic body radiation therapy in centrally and superiorly located stage I or isolated recurrent non-small-cell lung cancer. *Int J Radiat Oncol Biol Phys*, 2008, 72, 967-971.

[9] Lagerwaard, FJ; Haasbeek, CJ; Smit, EF; Slotman, BJ; Senan, S. Outcomes of risk-adapted fractionated stereotactic radiotherapy for stage I non-small-cell lung cancer. *Int J Radiat Oncol Biol Phys*, 2008, 70, 685-692.

[10] Stephans, KL; Djemil, T; Reddy, CA; et al. Comprehensive analysis of pulmonary function Test (PFT) changes after stereotactic body radiotherapy (SBRT) for stage I lung cancer in medically inoperable patients. *J Thorac Oncol*, 2009, 4, 838-844.

[11] Taremi, M; Hope, A; Dahele, M; et al. Stereotactic Body Radiotherapy for Medically Inoperable Lung Cancer: Prospective, Single-Center Study of 108 Consecutive Patients. *Int J Radiat Oncol Biol Phys*, 2011.

[12] Xia, T; Li, H; Sun, Q; et al. Promising clinical outcome of stereotactic body radiation therapy for patients with inoperable Stage I/II non-small-cell lung cancer. *Int J Radiat Oncol Biol Phys*, 2006, 66, 117-125.

[13] Song, SY; Choi, W; Shin, SS; et al. Fractionated stereotactic body radiation therapy for medically inoperable stage I lung cancer adjacent to central large bronchus. *Lung Cancer*, 2009, 66, 89-93.

[14] Guckenberger, M; Krieger, T; Richter, A; et al. Potential of image-guidance, gating and real-time tracking to improve accuracy in pulmonary stereotactic body radiotherapy. *Radiother Oncol*, 2009, 91, 288-295.

[15] Milano, MT; Chen, Y; Katz, AW; Philip, A; Schell, MC; Okunieff, P. Central thoracic lesions treated with hypofractionated stereotactic body radiotherapy. *Radiother Oncol*, 2009, 91, 301-306.

[16] Nuyttens JJ, van der Voort van Zyp NC, Praag J; et al. Outcome of four-dimensional stereotactic radiotherapy for centrally located lung tumors. *Radiother Onco,*. 2012, 102, 383-387.

In: The Revolution of Robotic …
Editor: Pierre-Yves Bondiau
ISBN: 978-1-62808-718-5

Chapter 12

CyberKnife Treatment for Stage III Lung Tumors

Pierre-Yves Bondiau[1,2*]
[1]Department of Radiation Oncology,
Antoine-Lacassagne Cancer Center, Nice, France
[2]University of Nice Sophia-Antipolis, Nice, France

Abstract

Patients with stage IIIA or IIIB lung cancer may benefit from high doses of irradiation, as we know that chemoradiotherapy can cause inoperable tumors to become operable and increase overall patient survival. For these patients, NSCLC could be sterilized when conventional techniques and fractionation schemes (2 Gy per fraction, 5 fractions per week) were used to deliver total radiation doses as high as 80-100 Gy. For patients who responding to chemoradiotherapy and those who have locoregional disease defined with CT and PET-CT, an increase of dose can be proposed, with a boost by Cyberknife. In this chapter, we will discuss the interest of SBRT used as a boost for locally advanced lung tumors.

* Email: pierre-yves.bondiau@nice.unicancer.fr.

Introduction

Lung cancer was virtually unknown at the beginning of the century, and it is now one of the most common cancers in France [1].

In contrast to other cancers that have a stable or declining frequency, the prevalence of lung cancer is rising. Its growth is related to smoking. Non-small cell lung cancer (NSCLC) is present in nonresectable but localized forms in 40% of NSCLC cases and is treated with surgery, chemotherapy, and radiotherapy. In France, lung cancer is increasing among women, but is stabilized in men. Lung cancer increased in women as a result of their increased smoking rates. A survey of the management of lung cancer in French hospitals [2] analyzed lesion distribution by TNM stage [3]. In this series of 5 667 patients, the breakdown of lesion staging is as follows:

Stage IA	4.8%
Stage IB	9.8%
Stage IIA	0.8%
Stage IIB	7.0%
Stage IIIA	14.1%
Stage IIIB	20.4%
Stage IV	42.6%

Lung cancer in locally advanced stages represented about 34.5% of all cases that were studied in this survey, a percentage which corresponds to the data in the international literature. Patient survival depends on the extent of the disease and thus the TNM stage; patients who have lesions with a lower TNM stage typically have a higher survival rate those who have lesions with a higher TNM stage. For example, this survey reported that 5-year survival rates for patients with stage I and II lesions were 67% and 38%, respectively.

The standard treatment for lung cancer is surgery. However, the primary curative intent approach for patients who refuse surgical resection or are determined by a multidisciplinary team to be inoperable continues to be primary radiation therapy.

Stereotactic body radiation therapy (SBRT) has increasingly been shown to provide greater local control than standard radiation therapy. And due to its benefit to stage II NSCLC, adjuvant chemotherapy is thus recommended, although it is not yet clear if adjuvant radiation or chemotherapy improves stage I NSCLC [4], stage IV benefit from chemotherapy.

Stage III lesions are heterogeneous. They are thus usually separated into stage IIIA (the stage where the lesion is potentially resectable and the role of neo-adjuvant therapy needs to be decided) and stage IIIB (for inoperable lesions that will be treated by chemoradiotherapy).

For patients with stage IIIA or IIIB disease, good performance scores, and minimal weight loss, treatment with a combination of chemotherapy and radiation (chemoradiotherapy) results in better survival than radiotherapy alone. Chemoradiotherapy can cause inoperable tumors to become operable and increase overall patient survival [5]. Fletcher et al. [6] showed that NSCLC could be sterilized when conventional techniques and fractionation schemes (2 Gy per fraction, 5 fractions per week) were used to deliver total radiation doses as high as 80-100 Gy. Wulf et al. [7] found that tumors could be controlled by 50% after receiving a biological equivalent dose (BED) of 94 Gy. Patients who respond to chemoradiotherapy and those who have locoregional disease (as demonstrated by CT and PET-CT) or have a stable disease may also benefit from high doses of irradiation. These patients can be treated with CyberKnife. However, some teams that use conventional radiation techniques consider a dose of 90.3 Gy to be intolerably toxic for healthy tissue (especially the lung and esophagus) [8].

When a typical radiochemotherapy (RCT) is made, concomitant chemotherapy prevents the total radiation dose from exceeding 66-70 Gy. In contrast, the current fractionation scheme that SBRT uses to exclusively treat early-stage primary lung cancer is 20-25 Gy per fraction with 3 fractions every 2 days. And although a total dose of 90.3 Gy seems to be the maximum dose that can be tolerated with conventional radiotherapy, this total can be safely exceeded with the use of SBRT and a stereotactic boost. A recent dosimetric evaluation [9] concluded that it is feasible to deliver chemoradiation (CRT) to 50.4 Gy and follow it with an SBRT boost to the primary tumor and involved regional lymph nodes with respect to normal tissue dose constraints.

In another study [10] 29 patients with locally advanced tumors were treated with conventional 3-dimensional conformal radiation therapy (3D-CRT) to the primary tumor and adjacent mediastinum. These patients received a total 3D-CRT dose of 45 Gy (25 fractions of 1.8 Gy each) within a 5-week period. After receiving this total dose, they then received an SBRT boost (3 fractions of 7.5 Gy each) to the PTV (10.7 Gy/fraction at the isocenter) within a 14-day period. The overall BED of the 3D-CRT and SBRT boost combination was calculated at 119.6 Gy. Results showed a 63% response rate (23% of the responses were complete and 40% of them were partial). The 3-year stage III cause-specific survival rate was 30%. The authors commented on SBRT's remarkably low toxicity rate (1.8%) and concluded that dose escalation seems to be an acceptable option for future clinical treatment.

Stage IIIA

However, tumor treatment is not always so straightforward. Some IIIB tumors can be operated on with good results after induction therapy (Gandara et al., 2003) and some IIIA tumors do not benefit from surgery (Suzuki et al., 1999). Late test results reported by the SWOG 88-05 trial (Albain et al., 1999) confirmed Gandara and Suzuki's findings. The SWOG trial found that IIIA (N2) and IIIB patients had similar 6-year survival rates of 20% and 22%, respectively, after induction therapy, chemoradiotherapy, and surgery. Most of the arguments that have been made regarding patient selection for neoadjuvant therapy and surgical resection provide evidence for a better prognosis but not for a beneficial impact of that treatment strategy. Furthermore, after consolidation chemotherapy or targeted therapy following definitive CRT, stage IIIA lesions have failed to improve. For patients who are preoperatively identified with stage IIIA NSCLC with discrete N2 involvement, definitive CRT therapy or induction therapy followed by surgery is recommended over surgery or radiation alone. However, these are the treatment recommendations for conventional radiotherapy.

SBRT has been used as a boost to the residual disease that remained after conventional radiotherapy, see figure 1 for an example of boost by Cyberknife. Feddock et al. [11] studied 17 patients with stage IIIA disease.

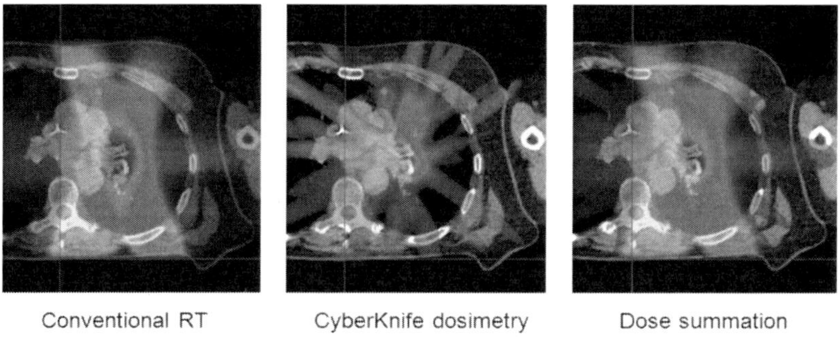

Figure 1. Example of a CyberKnife boost to stage IIIA lesions after conventional RT treatment of 46 Gy.

This use of SBRT did not lead to grade IV or V toxicity. Because the use of SBRT as a boost continues to be a novel approach in the management of this difficult disease, new randomized studies using SBRT boosts are needed.

Stage IIIB

Conventional RCT can significantly improve the local recurrence rate of stage IIIB lesions and also reduce the volume of some stage IIIB lung tumors. And using CyberKnife's robotic stereotactic radioablation (RSR) after RCT could deliver a boost of focused radiotherapy to lung tumors. Stage IIIB NSCLC is an advanced but not yet fully understood disease. Due to its superiority over other modalities, CRT is the most common way to treat stage IIIB NSCLC.

The lung team of Antoine Lacassagne cancer center conducted a monocentric phase I study with the goal of defining each patient's maximum tolerated dose. This upper limit was explored by first delivering 46 Gy in 23 fractions of 2 Gy of conventional RCT (using RCT cisplatin and docetaxel, as defined by Poudenx et al., in [12]) to NSCLC. RSR was then given in 3 fractions of 7-12 Gy to limited volumes (as defined by a CT scan) of residual NSCLC, see figure 2.

Using the time-to-event continual reassessment method, the amount of RSR that was given during each of the 6 levels was increased by 1 Gy per fraction. By using the linear quadratic equation to model doses of radiation therapy, we hypothesized that the combination of RCT and RSR would result in greater control of local NSCLC and achieve a minimum cumulative BED of approximately 84-142 Gy (depending of the level of the dose escalating study).

A total of 19 patients were treated between January 2010 and September 2012, see fig. 3 for an example of dosimetry. For levels 1, 2, 3, 4, 5, and 6, the number of patients was 3, 4, 2, 4, 3, and 3, respectively.

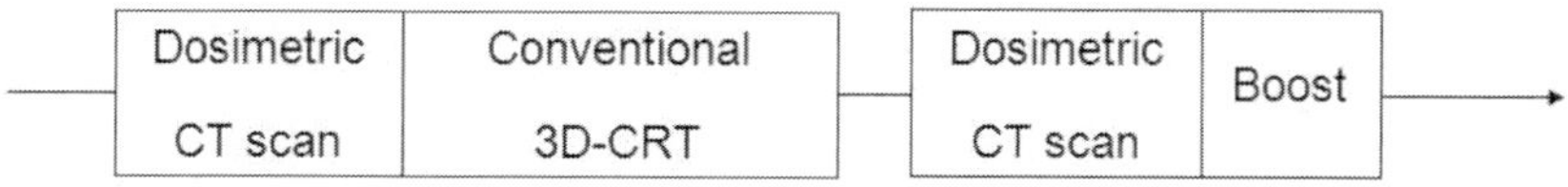

Figure 2. Example of SBRT boost after conventional 3D-CRT.

Toxicity was evaluated according to the Common Terminology Criteria for Adverse Events v3.0; grade 3-5 toxicities were considered limiting. With a median patient follow-up of 22 months (range, 0.5 to 32 months), the following grade 1 or 2 toxicities were reported (the number of affected patients is in parentheses): asthenia (11), alveolitis (11), cough (4), pleural effusion (4), pain (3), and heart failure (2). One patient who developed grade 3 esophagitis after receiving 46 Gy of conventional RCT later suffered grade 4 esophagitis (fistula) at level 5.

Our study concluded that patients who developed grade 3 toxicity after conventional RCT should not receive an RSR boost. This monocentric phase I study will be followed by a multicenter Phase II study.

Conclusion

For patients with a stage IIIA lung tumor, who also respond well to chemotherapy, a "closing" treatment with Cyberknife could be in their best interest.

For patients with a stage IIIB lung tumor, a boost with Cyberknife is feasible, with a low toxicity rate, but certain cases of an unexpected toxicity after conventional RT (>Gd II) must be discussed.

References

[1] Réseau des registres français de cancer http://www.invs.sante.fr/applications/cancers/estimations_regionales_1980_2005/donnees_generales.asp?region=93&nom_region=PACA

[2] *Rev Mal Respir.* 2002 Dec; 19(6):727-34. Epidemiologic of primary bronchial carcinoma management in the general French hospital centers. Blanchon F, Grivaux M, Collon T, Zureik M, Barbieux H, Bénichou-Flurin M, Breton JL, Coëtmeur D, Delclaux B, Asselain B, Piquet J.

[3] Revisions in the International System for Staging Lung Cancer. Mountain CF. *Chest.* 1997 Jun;111(6):1710-7.

[4] *Chest.* 2013 May;143(5 Suppl):e278S-313S. doi: 10.1378/chest.12-2359. *Treatment of Stage I and II Non-small Cell Lung Cancer: Diagnosis and Management of Lung Cancer*, 3rd ed: American College of Chest Physicians Evidence-Based Clinical Practice Guidelines.

[5] *J Clin Oncol.* 1999 Sep;17(9):2692-9. Phase III study of concurrent versus sequential thoracic radiotherapy in combination with mitomycin, vindesine, and cisplatin in unresectable stage III non-small-cell lung cancer. Furuse K, Fukuoka M, Kawahara M, Nishikawa H, Takada Y, Kudoh S, Katagami N, Ariyoshi Y.

[6] *Radiol Electrol Med Nucl.* 1972 Mar;53(3):201-6. Clinical dose-response curve of subclinical aggregates of epithelial cells. Fletcher GH.

[7] *Radiother Oncol.* 2005 Oct;77(1):83-7. Dose-response in stereotactic irradiation of lung tumors. Wulf J, Baier K, Mueller G, Flentje MP.

[8] Bradley J, Graham MV, Winter K, Purdy JA, Komaki R, Roa WH, Ryu JK, Bosch W, Emami B. Toxicity and outcome results of RTOG 9311: a phase I-II dose-escalation study using three-dimensional conformal radiotherapy in patients with inoperable non-small-cell lung carcinoma. *Int J Radiat Oncol Biol Phys.* 2005 Feb 1;61(2):318-28.

[9] *Front Oncol.* 2012;2:124. Dosimetric Feasibility of Dose Escalation Using SBRT Boost for Stage III Non-Small Cell Lung Cancer. Hepel JT, Peter J, Hiatt JR, Patel S, Osibanjo O, Safran H, Curran B, Dipetrillo T.

[10] *Int. J. Radiat Oncol Biol. Phys.* 2008 Nov 1;72(3):707-15. Once-weekly, high-dose stereotactic body radiotherapy for lung cancer: 6-year analysis of 60 early-stage, 42 locally advanced, and 7 metastatic lung cancers. Salazar OM, Sandhu TS, Lattin PB, Chang JH, Lee CK, Groshko GA, Lattin CJ.

[11] *Int. J. Radiation Oncol Biol Phys,* Vol. 85, No. 5, 1325e1331, 2013. Clinical Investigation: Thoracic Cancer Stereotactic Body Radiation Therapy Can Be Used Safelyto Boost Residual Disease in Locally Advanced Non-Small Cell Lung Cancer: A Prospective Study. J. Feddock, S. M. Arnold, B. J. Shelton,P. Sinha, G. Conrad,L. Chen, J. Rinehart, R. C. McGarry.

[12] *Oncology.* 2012;83(6):321-8. doi: 10.1159/000342081. Cisplatin-docetaxel induction plus concurrent 3-D conformal radiotherapy and weekly chemotherapy for locally advanced non-small cell lung cancer patients: a phase II trial. Poudenx M, Bondiau PY, Chamorey E, Venissac N, Otto J, Pourel N, Castelnau O, Tessier E, De Surmont Salasc B, Berdah JF, Pop D, Michel C, Mouroux J.

In: The Revolution of Robotic …
Editor: Pierre-Yves Bondiau
ISBN: 978-1-62808-718-5

Chapter 13

Stereotactic Ablative Re-Irradiation in Relapsed Non–Small Cell Lung Cancer

Jérôme Doyen[1,2*] and Pierre-Yves Bondiau[1,2†]
[1]Department of Radiation Oncology, Antoine-Lacassagne Cancer Center, Nice, France
[2]University of Nice Sophia-Antipolis, Nice, France

Abstract

Radiation treatment is often used in non operable localized non-small cell lung cancer with a good local control but some patients will present local relapse within or not far away from the original radiation field. To perform reirradiation in this setting with conventional radiotherapy will raise the problem of the toxicity in an organ at risk which already had received a substantial radiation dose. Thanks to new radiation techniques, namely stereotactic body radiotherapy, more precise treatment is possible reducing toxicity in organs at risk. This chapter will discuss the different available stereotactic body radiotherapy techniques and their clinical outcome, especially for toxicity and survival.

* Email: jerome.doyen@nice.unicancer.fr.
† Email: pierre-yves.bondiau@nice.unicancer.fr.

1. Introduction

1.1. The Role of Radiation Therapy in Non-Small Cell Lung Cancer

Radiation therapy plays an important role in the treatment of nonmetastatic non-small cell lung cancer (NSCLC).

Before the era of stereotactic body radiotherapy (SBRT), the above-mentioned tumors were treated with 3D conformal radiotherapy (3DRT) and standard fractionation (2 Gy per fraction). However, advances in SBRT devices now allow for more precise irradiation, increased dose per fraction (hypofractionation), and improved tumor control in stage I and II NSCLC. A retrospective analysis compared wedge resection with high dose SBRT in stage I NSCLS and showed comparable cause-specific survival [2]. In stage I and II NSCLCSBRT[2] had significantly better 3-year local control and overall survival (OS) results (at 90% and approximately 90%, respectively) than standard 3DRT (at approximately 75% and 70%[3], respectively). Due to findings such as these, SBRT has become the standard of care for the treatment of early and medically inoperable NSCLC.

1.2. Treatment Possibilities for Locally Relapsed NSCLC before the Era of SBRT

Many patients present nonmetastatic pulmonary relapse after surgery or radiotherapy. Indeed, local failure will be experienced by 53-69% of patients with locally advanced NSCLC that is treated with 3DRT and concomitant chemotherapy [4] and about 10% of patients that have early NSCLC that is treated with SBRT or surgery [2]. Estall et al., retrospectively analyzed 73 cases of relapsed NSCLC that were treated by a second course of irradiation between 1993 and 1996 [5]. The 3 years that were studied made it clear that their single-center experience irradiated NSCLC for a total of 527 patients. In other words, 13.8% of the patients who were irradiated for NSCLC were relapse patients, a percentage that is not unusual.

If the relapse site is solitary, some patients can elect for a second surgery (despite a mortality risk of 0-33% [6,7]). Conventional re-irradiation may also be feasible, but grade 3 toxicity rates have been reported in 0-26% of patients [8-12].

However, even if the recurrence is localized, it is very important to realize that patients cannot always be cured and might thus only be able to receive palliative treatment (such as by a lower re-irradiation dose). Palliative re-irradiation is mainly given to patients who have a poor general status and who are expected to have a higher rate of complications due to previous irradiation, the large size of the relapse, the number of nodules at relapse, and/or the proximity of organs at risk. The dose of re-irradiation can also vary depending on if the relapse is in-field or out-field (an out-field relapse is more suitable for curative re-irradiation).

Three-year survival rates range from 20-46% following a second lung resection [13, 14] and 47% following a salvage lung resection after irradiation [15]. Depending on the curative intent of the re-irradiation, the 2-year survival rate after re-irradiation ranges from 11-51% [9-12, 16]. High-dose re-irradiation SBRT can also be used as a salvage treatment in pulmonary tumors that were previously irradiated. Several groups have recently reported their experiences [17, 20]. Detailed results regarding outcomes and toxicities for second cancers resulting from conventional irradiation and SBRT re-irradiation can be found below.

1.3. The Problem of Normal Tissue Tolerance in the Re-irradiation Setting

Normal tissue tolerance to radiation was determined with (2 Gy per fraction). This tolerance is thus widely used to avoid an excessive risk of toxicities. When re-irradiation is used with conventional fractionated radiotherapy, these dose guidelines can be used to create a composite plan that can help predict toxicities. Some authors suggest that the longer the delay between irradiations, the higher the dose that can be prescribed. For acute-responding tissue, studies have demonstrated almost a complete recovery within a few months. Additionally, De Crevoisier et al., reported that the number of grade 3 incidents of mucositis and dermatitis was the same for either a primary or secondary irradiation setting [21]. Whether or not late-responding tissue recovers depends on the specific organ at risk; most tissues seem to at least partially recover. For example, an excessive rate of osteoradionecrosis of the mandible during the re-irradiation of head and neck appears at 135 Gy, a dose that is much higher than what it is recommended by normal tissue complication probability guidelines [22]. One must be very careful when re-irradiating lung tumors due to the facts that the lungs can recover from disease that is in the acute phase but recover less successfully for late fibrosis. Furthermore, most studies show a cumulative toxic effect in patients who undergo multiple irradiations. The spinal cord in animal models might also recover from irradiation (approximately 61% several years after 44 Gy [23]). In humans no recovery seems to exist for the heart, bladder, and kidney; these organs thus need to be carefully spared during re-irradiation [24].

Because composite treatment planning is very difficult to construct, applying very high doses in the re-irradiation setting (as is the case with SBRT is very complex. This complexity results from the fact that the dose per fraction is very different between the first and second course of irradiation. Some authors have also found that the linear-quadratic model is no longer valid when the dose per fraction exceeds 6-8 Gy (which very often occurs when SBRT is used) [25]. Additional research is needed for composite treatment planning.

2. Toxicities and Outcomes after Conventional Re-irradiation to the Localized Relapse of NSCLC

The toxicities and outcomes that follow conventional re-irradiation to the localized relapse of NSCLC is a topic that has been recently and extensively reviewed by others [26]. Conventional re-irradiation refers to re-irradiation that uses fractions of 2-3 Gy.

To summarize, the studies that have reported on this topic included few patients and heterogeneous doses. Variations were also found in treatment schedules, including the use of different definitions for the gross target volume (GTV) and clinical target volume (CTV), types of relapse, histologic types (sometimes including small cell lung cancer patients), and stages of disease (from stages I to IV). These differences make it very difficult to assert strong conclusions regarding the outcomes of conventional re-irradiation. Also, these studies were retrospective and only a few of them were prospective Phase I, II, or III trials. Only Wu et al., and Kramer et al., have performed a prospective Phase I-II trial in this setting [8, 12].

2.1. Patient and Treatment Characteristics in Studies that Reported on Conventional Re-irradiation

These studies involved 19 to 44 patients [9, 27]. Because, as previously detailed in Section I.b., the dose amount depended on whether the re-irradiation treatment intended to cure or palliate, re-irradiation doses ranged from 6 Gy [28] -70 Gy [9]. Initial dose also greatly varied and ranged from 25-80 Gy [9, 29].

2.2. Toxicities after Conventional Re-irradiation

The typical toxicities that follow conventional re-irradiation are rib fracture (0-3%), pneumonitis (0-35%) (1 study reported fatal pneumonitis in 4% of its participants [29]), myelopathy (0-5%), and esophagitis (0-77%) (reviewed by Jeremic et al. [26]). A higher rate of toxicity was observed in a study by Okamoto et al. They used the highest dose at the first or second course of irradiation (median cumulative dose of 110-150 Gy) [9] and reported Grade 3 and 4 esophagitis in 21% of their participants and grade 2 acute pneumonitis in 35% of them. The study with the highest toxicity rate was a prospective Phase I-II trial conducted by Wu et al. [12]. This study reported that 26% of its population had late grade 2-3 lung fibrosis. Authors of this study raise the point that we often underestimate treatment side-effects when they are reported in a retrospective versus a prospective manner.

2.3. Response and Survival after Conventional Re-irradiation

Symptoms greatly improved after a second course of radiotherapy. Improvements were found in hemoptysis, cough, chest pain, and dyspnea in 33-100%, 50-77%, 40-80%, and 35-100% of cases, respectively. Symptoms globally improved at a rate of 70-80% al. [26].

OS at one year ranged from 8.7-59% [12, 30]. These rate differences are largely again due to the different inclusion criteria that each study used. Wu et al., reported the highest 1-year OS rate (59%). This high rate is perhaps due to the fact that all of the study participants were Phase I-II trial patients who had relapsed more than 6 months after their first irradiation, had a Karnosfky performance status of $\geq$ 70, and exhibited a forced expiratory volume of 1 s >

1 L. The Wu et al., study patients also received a high re-irradiation dose of 46-60 Gy [12].

Prognostic factors for better survival were rarely analyzed in these studies. However, Tada et al. [11] and Cetingoz et al. [30] found that a longer interval (up to approximately 1 year) between irradiation treatments may confer better survival. Although dose response was rarely studied and rigorous comparisons cannot be made, we can conjecture that studies with the highest re-irradiation doses may have the highest overall survival rates [9, 12].

In conclusion, re-irradiation with conventional radiotherapy is feasible. An improved OS seems to be reached with a higher re-irradiation dose, but this higher dose can increase the rate of grade 2-3 pneumonitis. This toxicity rate supports the rationale for using SBRT to re-irradiate relapsed lung tumors.

3. Toxicities and Outcomes after SBRT Re-irradiation in the Localized Relapse of NSCLC

3.1. SBRT Techniques

SBRT can be performed by several techniques that can greatly differ. They can vary not only because of the procedure itself, but also due to differences in the size of the final planned target volume (PTV) and the given dose per fraction. Although this section does not provide an exhaustive listing, it aims to describe some of the methods available for re-irradiation.

One SBRT method is non–image guided SBRT. Peulen et al. [18] treated 29 patients according to the following procedure. After the GTV was delineated on the CT-scan, a margin of 5-10 mm was applied to define the CTV and further expanded by approximately 10 mm for the PTV. Abdominal compression was used if movement due to respiration (as evaluated by fluoroscopy) exceeded 10 mm. Five to 10 coplanar multileaf collimator beams were used. The prescribed dose in the re-irradiation setting was about 2-3 fractions of 15 Gy or 5 fractions of 8 Gy.

Another way to use SBRT is with inter-fraction image-guided SBRT. Kelly et al. [19] (MD Anderson, Texas, USA) treated 37 patients with the following technique. After a four-dimensional (4D) computed tomography (CT) scan was taken, a GTV was obtained that corresponded to the sum of the GTV of each phase of the 4D-CT (the internal GTV). The CTV was then created by an automatic 8-mm expansion and the PTV was made up of an additional expansion of 3 mm. Although the tumor was not tracked during the procedure, orthogonal port films tracked it before the procedure at every fraction (inter-fraction, image- guided SBRT). Six to 9 beams (sometimes noncoplanar) were used. The prescribed dose was about 50 Gy in 4 fractions.

The last SBRT option that this chapter will discuss is intra-fraction image-guided SBRT. This technique was used by both Coon et al. [20] in 12 patients and the anticancer center of Nice, France (Centre Antoine-Lacassagne) in 19 patients [31].

This technique is sometimes referred to as "robotic" SBRT (rSBRT). It is characterized by image-guided and real-time repositioning of the treatment beam during the irradiation session. This repositioning is made possible by the gold fiducial(s) that is implanted into the tumor; the implantation technique has been previously well documented [32, 33]. Soon after the gold fiducial is implanted, the planning CT scan is realized. After the GTV is delineated, the CTV is obtained through an automatic 5 mm expansion. An additional 1 (upper tumors) to 2 mm (lower tumors) expansion is used to define the PTV. Respiration movements are continuously registered during the treatment and correlate with the position of the gold fiducial (using orthogonal port film), thus enabling the real-time tracking of the tumor.

Approximately 100 to 250 noncoplanar beams are usually used and the prescribed dose ranges from 60 Gy in 3 fractions (peripheral tumors) to 50-60 Gy in 5 fractions (central tumors).

3.2. Toxicities after SABR Re-irradiation

Toxicities greatly varied between the 4 studies that studied the different SBRT techniques. Specifically, the Kelly et al. [19] and Peulen et al. [18] experiences reported grade 3 toxicities (pneumonitis, esophagitis, skin ulcer, and cough) at a rate of 33% and 37.9%, respectively. Kelly et al., did not report any toxic death while Peulen et al., reported 3 cases of massive hemoptysis, each occurring at a median follow-up of 4 months after re-irradiation. The Coon et al., [20] and Bondiau et al. [31] studies that used rSBRT did not report any grade 3 toxicities. In the latter study, one patient died of massive hemoptysis after the study was published (11 months after the patient was re-irradiated). This patient had a previous history of hemoptysis at the diagnosis of relapse. When the patient died, however, the previous CT evaluation found no evidence of relapse.

This patient received one of the lowest re-irradiation doses (45 Gy), but the tumor was near great vessels. The Bondiau et al., experience found that the most common grade 1-2 toxicities were nonsymptomatic alveolitis (58%), pain (26.3%), esophagitis (21%), and asthenia (21%) [31]. This toxicity profile was very similar to was what reported by Kelly et al. [19].

Although the Kelly et al. [19], Peulen et al. [18], and Bondiau et al. [31] experiences all had a similar median follow-up (15, 12, and 16 months, respectively) and a similar median irradiation dose (50 Gy in 4 fractions, 40 Gy in 4 fractions, and 60 Gy in 3-5 fractions, respectively), the toxicity profile of rSBRT re-irradiation may be somewhat more favorable. Specifically, when rSBRT was used there was 1 grade 3-5 (3.5%, 1/28 patients) toxicity as compared to a grade 3-5 toxicity rate of 33% (12/36 patients) and 37.9% (11/29 patients), respectively. However, these SBRT re-irradiation studies cannot be rigorously compared to each other for the same reasons as those of the conventional re-irradiation studies. That is, each SBRT study reported on heterogeneous patient tumors and treatment schedules. Nevertheless, as compared to other techniques, we might at least conjecture that rSBRT could deliver a higher re-irradiation dose without a higher toxicity rate.

As bleeding is the major limiting toxicity, physicians need to be very careful when they prescribe SBRT re-irradiation treatment to patients with central tumors that are next to big vessels (especially if hemoptysis is present during re-irradiation). It seems that big vessels (as well as the heart) do not recover completely, or even partially, after their first curative irradiation.

When given 3 or 5 fractions of re-irradiation SBRT, dose constraints to big vessels are about 39 or 47 Gy to 10 cc, respectively [34]. Although these vessels previously received a conventional dose of 60-66 Gy, this constraint must be greatly lowered in order to be more conservative. This constraint may need to be less than 20 Gy, but its threshold is still being determined.

Another group updated the experience of the MD Anderson radiation department and found multiple predictors of severe (> grade 2) pneumonitis: a poor general status (a performance status of 2-3), an FEV 1 of ≤ 65%, a previous PTV spanning the bilateral mediastinum, and a V20 ≥ of 30% on the composite plan (previous radiotherapy + SBRT) [35].

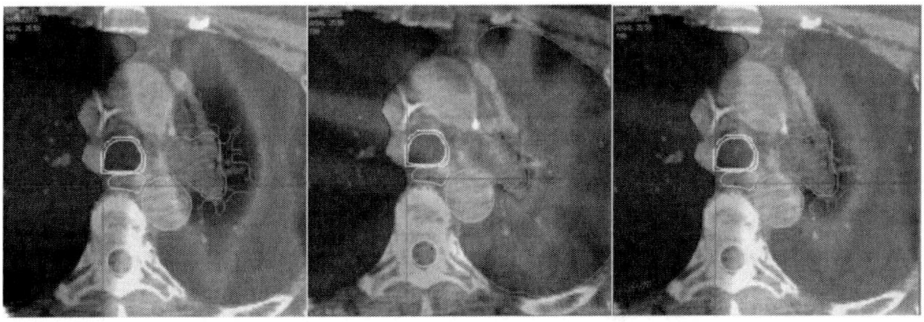

Figure 1. Example of dose summation for re-irradiation treatment. Left: dose delivered with conventional 3DRT. Middle: dose delivered with CyberKnife. Summation of 3DRT and Cyberknife doses.

3.3. Response and Survival after SBRT Re-irradiation

Not all of the SBRT re-irradiation studies reported whether or not symptoms improved. This absence may be due to the facts that SBRT is commonly and intuitively prescribed to patients with a very limited relapse. Additionally, most of the study patients were not symptomatic.

Kelly et al. [19] reported a 100% rate of response while the response to our experience was reached in 50% of patients (data not published), and the stabilization rate was35.7% leading to clinical benefit (response + stabilization) in 85.7%.

Bondiau et al. reported a 1-year OS rate of about 67.3% and a 1-year local control rate of 75.1% (data not published). These outcomes were similar to those of the Kelly et al., experience [19] (which reported a 1-year OS rate of 85% and local control rate of 92%). Both studies reported low progression-free survival and at 2 years it was only 22.7% (Bondiau et al) and 26% (Kelly et al).

Our survival rate seems to be better than that of conventional re-irradiation (which has a 1-year OS between 8.7-59%) but, again, selection bias and confounding factors could strongly impair such a comparison.

Conclusion

In summary, re-irradiation with conventional radiotherapy is feasible and an improved OS seems to be reached with a higher re-irradiation dose but with an increased rate of grade 2-3 pneumonitis. Recent advances in radiation technology have resulted in SBRT, a technique in which much higher hypofractionated doses are delivered to tumors while normal tissue irradiation is dramatically decreased. As compared with conventional re-irradiation, SBRT might improve local tumor control and OS. The rate of distant progression with SBRT re-irradiation, however, is still very high (approximately 70% at 2 years) and the improvement of subsequent systemic treatments (i.e., chemotherapy) remains the greatest challenge in treating relapsed NSCLC.

More homogenous prospective Phase II trials are needed in order to better identify patients who might benefit from very high re-irradiation doses. These patients could include those who have had an interval of more than 12 months between 2 radiation treatments and who qualify for the highest dose (i.e., patients with good performance status and no history of hemoptysis or major vessel irradiation). However, as a conventional re-irradiation schedule can still improve symptoms by 70-80%, this treatment could be offered to patients who do not qualify for the Phase II trials.

References

[1] Alberts WM: Diagnosis and management of lung cancer executive summary: ACCP evidence-based clinical practice guidelines (2nd Edition). *Chest* 132:1S-19S, 2007.

[2] Grills IS, Mangona VS, Welsh R, et al.: Outcomes after stereotactic lung radiotherapy or wedge resection for stage I non-small-cell lung cancer. *J Clin Oncol* 28:928-35, 2010.

[3] Fang LC, Komaki R, Allen P, et al.: Comparison of outcomes for patients with medically inoperable Stage I non-small-cell lung cancer treated with two-dimensional vs. three-dimensional radiotherapy. *Int J Radiat Oncol Biol Phys* 66:108-16, 2006.

[4] Fournel P, Robinet G, Thomas P, et al.: Randomized phase III trial of sequential chemoradiotherapy compared with concurrent chemoradiotherapy in locally advanced non-small-cell lung cancer:

Groupe Lyon-Saint-Etienne d'Oncologie Thoracique-Groupe Francais de Pneumo-Cancerologie NPC 95-01 Study. *J Clin Oncol* 23:5910-7, 2005.

[5] Estall V, Barton MB, Vinod SK: Patterns of radiotherapy re-treatment in patients with lung cancer: a retrospective, longitudinal study. *J Thorac Oncol* 2:531-6, 2007.

[6] Levasseur P, Regnard JF, Icard P, et al.: Cancer surgery on a single residual lung. *Eur J Cardiothorac Surg* 6:639-40; discussion 641, 1992.

[7] Terzi A, Furlan G, Gorla A, et al.: Lung resection on single residual lung after pneumonectomy for bronchogenic carcinoma. *Thorac Cardiovasc Surg* 45:273-6, 1997.

[8] Kramer GW, Gans S, Ullmann E, et al.: Hypofractionated external beam radiotherapy as retreatment for symptomatic non-small-cell lung carcinoma: an effective treatment? *Int J Radiat Oncol Biol Phys* 58:1388-93, 2004.

[9] Okamoto Y, Murakami M, Yoden E, et al.: Reirradiation for locally recurrent lung cancer previously treated with radiation therapy. *Int J Radiat Oncol Biol Phys* 52:390-6, 2002.

[10] Poltinnikov IM, Fallon K, Xiao Y, et al.: Combination of longitudinal and circumferential three-dimensional esophageal dose distribution predicts acute esophagitis in hypofractionated reirradiation of patients with non-small-cell lung cancer treated in stereotactic body frame. *Int J Radiat Oncol Biol Phys* 62:652-8, 2005.

[11] Tada T, Fukuda H, Matsui K, et al.: Non-small-cell lung cancer: reirradiation for loco-regional relapse previously treated with radiation therapy. *Int J Clin Oncol* 10:247-50, 2005.

[12] Wu KL, Jiang GL, Qian H, et al.: Three-dimensional conformal radiotherapy for locoregionally recurrent lung carcinoma after external beam irradiation: a prospective phase I-II clinical trial. *Int J Radiat Oncol Biol Phys* 57:1345-50, 2003.

[13] Spaggiari L, Grunenwald D, Girard P, et al.: Cancer resection on the residual lung after pneumonectomy for bronchogenic carcinoma. *Ann Thorac Surg* 62:1598-602, 1996.

[14] Westermann CJ, van Swieten HA, Brutel de la Riviere A, et al.: Pulmonary resection after pneumonectomy in patients with bronchogenic carcinoma. *J Thorac Cardiovasc Surg* 106:868-74, 1993.

[15] Bauman JE, Mulligan MS, Martins RG, et al.: Salvage lung resection after definitive radiation (>59 Gy) for non-small cell lung cancer: surgical and oncologic outcomes. *Ann Thorac Surg* 86:1632-8; discussion 1638-9, 2008.

[16] Hauswald H, Stoiber E, Rochet N, et al.: Treatment of recurrent bronchial carcinoma: the role of high-dose-rate endoluminal brachytherapy. *Int J Radiat Oncol Biol Phys* 77:373-7, 2010.

[17] Dworzecki T, Idasiak A, Sygula D, et al.: Stereotactic radiotherapy (SBRT) as a sole or salvage therapy in non-small cell lung cancer patients. *Neoplasma* 59:114-20, 2012.

[18] Peulen H, Karlsson K, Lindberg K, et al.: Toxicity after reirradiation of pulmonary tumours with stereotactic body radiotherapy. *Radiother Oncol* 101:260-6, 2011.

[19] Kelly P, Balter PA, Rebueno N, et al.: Stereotactic body radiation therapy for patients with lung cancer previously treated with thoracic radiation. *Int J Radiat Oncol Biol Phys* 78:1387-93, 2010.

[20] Coon D, Gokhale AS, Burton SA, et al.: Fractionated stereotactic body radiation therapy in the treatment of primary, recurrent, and metastatic lung tumors: the role of positron emission tomography/computed tomography-based treatment planning. *Clin Lung Cancer* 9:217-21, 2008.

[21] De Crevoisier R, Bourhis J, Domenge C, et al.: Full-dose reirradiation for unresectable head and neck carcinoma: experience at the Gustave-Roussy Institute in a series of 169 patients. *J Clin Oncol* 16:3556-62, 1998.

[22] Salama JK, Vokes EE, Chmura SJ, et al.: Long-term outcome of concurrent chemotherapy and reirradiation for recurrent and second primary head-and-neck squamous cell carcinoma. *Int J Radiat Oncol Biol Phys* 64:382-91, 2006.

[23] Ang KK, Jiang GL, Feng Y, et al.: Extent and kinetics of recovery of occult spinal cord injury. *Int J Radiat Oncol Biol Phys* 50:1013-20, 2001.

[24] Mantel F, Flentje M, Guckenberger M: Stereotactic body radiation therapy in the re-irradiation situation - a review. Radiat Oncol 8:7, 2013.

[25] Astrahan M: Some implications of linear-quadratic-linear radiation dose-response with regard to hypofractionation. *Med Phys* 35:4161-72, 2008.

[26] Jeremic B, Videtic GM: Chest reirradiation with external beam radiotherapy for locally recurrent non-small-cell lung cancer: a review. *Int J Radiat Oncol Biol Phys* 80:969-77, 2011.

[27] Ebara T, Tanio N, Etoh T, et al.: Palliative re-irradiation for in-field recurrence after definitive radiotherapy in patients with primary lung cancer. *Anticancer Res* 27:531-4, 2007.

[28] Green N, Melbye RW: Lung cancer: retreatment of local recurrence after definitive irradiation. *Cancer* 49:865-8, 1982.

[29] Gressen EL, Werner-Wasik M, Cohn J, et al.: Thoracic reirradiation for symptomatic relief after prior radiotherapeutic management for lung cancer. *Am J Clin Oncol* 23:160-3, 2000.

[30] Cetingoz R, Arican-Alicikus Z, Nur-Demiral A, et al.: Is re-irradiation effective in symptomatic local recurrence of non small cell lung cancer patients? A single institution experience and review of the literature. *J BUON* 14:33-40, 2009.

[31] Bondiau PY, Doyen J, Mammar H, et al.: [Reirradiation of spine and lung tumor with CyberKnife]. *Cancer Radiother* 14:438-41, 2010.

[32] Bondiau PY, Benezery K, Beckendorf V, et al.: [CyberKnife robotic stereotactic radiotherapy: technical aspects and medical indications]. *Cancer Radiother* 11:338-44, 2007.

[33] Whyte RI, Crownover R, Murphy MJ, et al.: Stereotactic radiosurgery for lung tumors: preliminary report of a phase I trial. *Ann Thorac Surg* 75:1097-101, 2003.

[34] Benedict SH, Yenice KM, Followill D, et al.: Stereotactic body radiation therapy: the report of AAPM Task Group 101. *Med Phys* 37:4078-101, 2010.

[35] Liu H, Zhang X, Vinogradskiy YY, et al.: Predicting radiation pneumonitis after stereotactic ablative radiation therapy in patients previously treated with conventional thoracic radiation therapy. *Int J Radiat Oncol Biol Phys* 84:1017-23, 2012.

In: The Revolution of Robotic …
Editor: Pierre-Yves Bondiau
ISBN: 978-1-62808-718-5

Chapter 14

Treatment of Lung Metastasis

Joost Jan Nuyttens[1,*], Juliette Van Loon[1] and Pierre-Yves Bondiau[2,3]

[1]Department of Radiation Oncology, Erasmus MC-Daniel den Hoed Cancer Center, Rotterdam, the Netherlands
[2]Department of Radiation Oncology, Antoine-Lacassagne Cancer Center, Nice, France
[3]University of Nice Sophia-Antipolis, Nice, France

Abstract

The CyberKnife provides the advantage of allowing fractionated treatment to multiple secondary tumors. This chapter will present the results of published data on this indication. The delivery of precisely targeted radiation doses to secondary lung tumors in a hypofractionated fashion is feasible and safe. Image-guided robotic stereotactic radiosurgery of pulmonary metastases with the CyberKnife achieves good rates of local disease control.

The toxicity is limited to the surrounding tissues. In cases of slow growing cancer, SBRT for solitary or oligometastatic tumors may be beneficial for patients.

* Email : j.nuyttens@erasmusmc.nl.

Introduction

The tumor-ablative effects of high-dose stereotactic body radiation therapy (SBRT) for lung cancer can be safely extended to metastatic lesions. Published SBRT studies with the use of the CyberKnife include a very small number of patients, but have shown that delivering lower doses of SBRT can locally control the metastasis. However, the doses that are often used to treat metastatic lung lesions are the same as those for primary lesions.

Colorectal cancer it is the most common origin of pulmonary metastases. It is often a slow growing primary cancer with lung metastases for which treatment by Robotic SBRT can be offered.

In this chapter we analyze our CyberKnife databank to present the results obtained after the treatment of pulmonary metastases of colorectal primary tumors with the CyberKnife.

Patients and Methods

From January 1st, 2007 to December 31st, 2012, sixty-nine metastases were treated with the CyberKnife in 36 patients (22 men, 12 women) average of 1.9 metastasis by patient. The minimal number of metastasis was 1 and the maximal number was seven, treated over a time period of three years. The average patient age was 63 years [med: 64, min: 34, max: 78] at diagnosis.

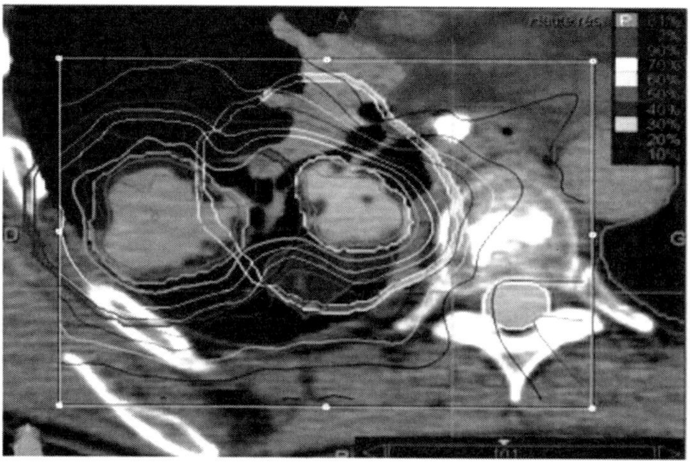

Figure 1. Two lung metastasis treated in the same time.

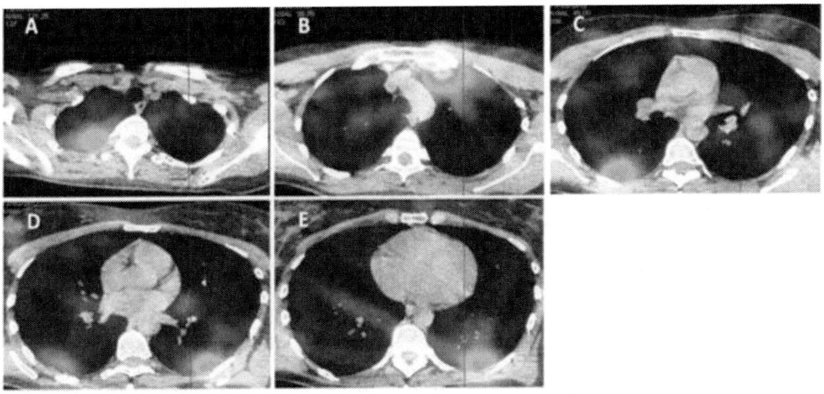

Figure 2. Treatment of five lung metastasis. A: right upper lobe metastasis. B: Left upper lobe metastasis.C: right lower lobe metastasis. D: left lower lobe metastasis 1.E : left lower lobe metastasis 2.

The maximum number of metastases treated at the same time was 2 (see figure 1). The maximum metastases treated consecutively was 5 (see figure 2). For dose summation we used specific software developed by Aquilab (http://www. aquilab.com/en).

Patients received an initial treatment including: 32 patients underwent surgery on the primary tumor, 24 patients received adjuvant chemotherapy and ten patients received chemoradiation treatment or radiation treatment alone. Thirty patients underwent a PET/CT in the initial evaluation. Ten patients had one or more secondary locations in other organs [liver: 9, bone: 1, adrenal gland: 1]. Among the comorbidities we noticed: 2 myocardial infarction, 8 heart failure, 15 arterial disease, 2 stroke, 1 hemiplegia, 3 diabetes, 7 emphysema, 2 second cancer and 6 renal failure. The average time of metastasis onset after the initial diagnosis was 33 months [med: 31, min: 0, max: 123]. Treatment of lung metastases did include: chemotherapy (18), surgery (14) and radiotherapy (5). In average, there were 2 different chemotherapy protocols given before the start of the stereotactic radiotherapy treatment [med: 2, min: 1 max: 4].

Results

An average of three lung metastases were treated with stereotactic radiotherapy [med: 3 min: 1 max: 6]. In average, one fiducial [med: 1 min: 0, max: 3] was placed.

Table 1. Local control in published studies

author	year	patients	complication	local control at 3-9 months
Coon [1]	2008	12	na	62%
Castelli [2]	2008	4	0	100%
Swangsilpa [3]	2013	6	na	75%

na: not available.

Complications related to the placement of fiducials for the 69 radiotherapy treatments was pneumothorax (7) and migration of the fiducial (1).

The median dose was 60 Gy [mean: 54, min: 20, max: 75] in 3 fractions [med: 3 min: 1 max: 5]. The average diameter of the GTV was 18 mm [med: 14, min: 2 max: 87]. The location of the metastasis was peripheral in 42 cases.

The median follow-up was 21 months [med: 17, min: 3, max: 60].

Of the 69 treatments, there were four local recurrences (5%) occurring on average 40 months after treatment with CyberKnife [med: 44, min: 20, max: 53].

Of the 36 patients, 5 died of tumor progression: cerebral metastasis (2), bleeding (1), carcinomatous lymphangitis (1).

Toxicity

Previous studies do not report an increase of toxicity with CyberKnife treatment for the lung metastasis compared to the stereotactic radiotherapy treatment of primary early stage lung tumors. These results can be anticipated as the doses are the same for both tumors. Furthermore, some teams reduce the margin from the Clinical Target Volume to the Planning Targer Volume to zero (Cf. Annex B) to decrease the risk of lung toxicity. Lung toxicity can appear if multiple lung metastasis are treated. In our experience, we don't treat more than 3 metastases in one lung (maximum 6 for the two lungs, depending on the volume of the mets) in order to avoid lung toxicity (Cf. Figure 1, 2).

Conclusion

Stereotactic radiotherapy with the CyberKnife for lung metastasis appears to be a safe and efficient treatment, it can be proposed for a patient presenting a small number of metastases, up to three localized in the lung in our experience. Local control seems to be excellent in our experience. Toxicity is acceptable, as it is in the stereotactic treatment of the early stage lung cancer.

References

[1] Coon D, Gokhale AS, Burton SA, Heron DE, Ozhasoglu C, Christie N. Fractionated stereotactic body radiation therapy in the treatment of primary, recurrent, and metastatic lung tumors: the role of positron emission tomography/computed tomography-based treatment planning. *Clin. Lung Cancer*. 2008 Jul; 9(4):217-21.

[2] Castelli J, Thariat J, Benezery K, Padovani B, Ducreux D, Venissac N, Poudenx M, Otto J, Mouroux J, Bondiau PY. *Cancer Radiother*. 2008 Dec; 12(8): 793-9. [Feasibility and efficacy of cyberknife radiotherapy for lung cancer: early results].

[3] Swangsilpa T, Yongvithisatid P, Pairat K, Dechsupa P, Dhanachai M, Dangprasert S, Narkwong L, Sitathanee C, Puataweepong P, Puddhikarant P, Jiarpinitnun C, Witoonpanich P, Ruangkanchanasetr R, Ukhumpun T, Khaophong J. Preliminary experience of CyberKnife treatment of lung metastasis: the question about real clinical benefit. *J. Med. Assoc. Thai.* 2013 May; 96(5): 603-13.

In: The Revolution of Robotic …
Editor: Pierre-Yves Bondiau
ISBN: 978-1-62808-718-5

Chapter 15

Toxicity Outcomes in Studies of the Stereotactic Radiotherapy of Lung Tumors

Axel Leysalle[1,2*] and Pierre-Yves Bondiau[1,2]
[1]Department of Radiation Oncology, Antoine-Lacassagne Cancer Center, Nice, France
[2]University of Nice Sophia-Antipolis, Nice, France

Abstract

Retrospective and prospective studies published in the past decade have established the feasibility, safety, and efficacy of SBRT in these patients using a variety of dose regimens and technologies. There is now a large literature with dosimetric correlation to toxicities of various organs in the literature. This chapter reviews clinical studies investigating normal tissue constraints for ablative radiation dose range based on studies with dosimetric parameters correlating with toxicities in the literature for lung tumors.

[*] Corresponding author: Email: axel.leysalle@nice.unicancer.fr.

I. Introduction

In this chapter we summarize common toxicities that can result from the delivery of stereotactic body radiation therapy (SBRT) treatment to the lungs. These toxicities include radiation pneumonitis, bronchial stenosis or necrosis, rib fracture, skin toxicity, oesophageal injury, and injury to the brachial plexus. SBRT-related toxicities are usually modest, with 3-10% of patients reporting grade $\geq$ 3 toxicity (according to the Common Terminology Criteria for Adverse Events). The extent of these toxicities depends on the tumors, dose regimens, and delivery system characteristics [1].

3D-SBRT, three-dimensional stereotactic radiation therapy; 4D-CT, four-dimensional computed tomography planning scan; COPD, chronic obstructive pulmonary disease; CW, chest wall; IMRT, intensity-modulated radiotherapy; NCICTC, National Cancer Institute Common Toxicity Criteria; OBI, on-board imaging; Pgrade, pathological grade; PS, performance status; RTS, respiration tracking system; SBF, stereotactic body frame.

II. Lung

Radiation pneumonitis (RP) has always been a critical concern for oncologists that treat non–small cell lung cancer (NSCLC). RP also becomes more complex when SBRT is used. SBRT treatment to the lung also causes the risk of developing symptomatic pneumonitis to be 9.4-28% [8, 16, 24, 34-45]. However, symptoms that are attributed to SBRT may actually be overestimated due to their being combined with exacerbations of chronic obstructive pulmonary disease (COPD) and cases of pneumonia. Although SBRT has been associated with a small decrease in lung function, it is important to note that a greater loss of lung function was observed in patients that had better pulmonary functioning at baseline [46]. In general, for to most of patients that are treated with SBRT lung function decreased slightly or not at all [47, 48].

Table 1. Summary of studies with reported toxicity

Study	nbr	Dose/fraction	Immbolisation of image guidance	Median follow-up	toxicity
Baumann et al. [2]	138	48-30 Gy/2-4	3D SRT Body Frame Fluoroscopy	33	Grade 3–4: 10.1%
Baumann et al. [3]	57	45 Gy/3	SBF	15,3	Grade 3–4: 28%; dyspnea, fibrosis, heart failure, and rib fracture
Fakiris et al. [4]	70	60-66 Gy/3	SBF, vacuum pillow, abdominal compression	50,2	Grade 3–5: 17.1%: Peripheral lesions: 10.4%; central lesions: 27.3% Grade 5: 4 bacterial pneumonia, 1 pericardial effusion, 1 massive hemoptysis (last 2 with central tumors)
Kopek et al. [5]					Grade 3–4: 14%
Koto et al. [6]	31	45 Gy/3	half-body vacuum cast, active breathing control, 3D SRT	32	NCI-CTC 3.0 Grade 3 pneumonitis: 1.1%
Nagata et al. [7]	45	48 Gy	SBF, vacuum, 3D SRT	30	NCI-CTC 2.0 No >grade 3 toxicity after median follow-up of 30 months
Onishi et al. [8]	257	18-75 Gy/ 1-22	NA	38	NCI-CTC 2.0 >Grade 2 pneumonitis: 5.4% Grade 3 esophagitis: 0.8% Grade 3–4 dermatitis: 1.2% (tumor close to chest wall) Ribe fracture 4
Salazar et al. [9]	102	40 Gy/4 22.5 Gy/3 for a boost after 45 Gy	diaphragmatic press, external fiducial markers, active breathing control	38	Only 3% with grade 2 toxicity (no >grade 2 toxicity) 2 Symptomatic pneumonitis 1 Severe symptomatic fibrosis and sustained dyspnea in the treated lung

Table 1. (Continued)

Study	nbr	Dose/fraction	Immbolisation of image guidance	Median follow-up	toxicity
Takeda et al. [10]	63	50 Gy/5	Vac-Lok immobilization system	31	Radiation pneumonitis: 3 patients 1 Grade 2, 2 grade 3 (1/2 later developed bacterial pneumonia)
Uematsu et al. [11]	131	50-60 Gy/5-6		36	1 Grade 5: broncho-left pulmonary vein fistula 2 grade 2 pneumonitis 3 Patients with minor bone fracture 20% Complained of chest pain, no treatment needed
Chang et al. [12]	130	50 Gy/4	4DCT Vac-LOK cradle	26	4 Grade 2 pneumonitis all in recurrent tumors Grade 2–3 dermatitis and chest wall pain in 3 pts who received >35 Gy to the skin and ribs Brachial plexus neuropathy in 1 patient who received 40 Gy to a large area
Collins et al. [13]	21	42–60 Gy/3	CyberKnife, RTS		Acute grade 3 pneumonitis in 1 patient who received 60 Gy + Tarceva
Fritz et al. [14]	40	30 Gy/1	4D-CT OBI	20	Grade 4 rib fracture 5%, 62 toxicity otherwise
Hoyer et al. [15]	40	45 Gy/3	stereotactic body frame abdominal compression		Progression to Pgrade 2 toxicity in 48% of patients Only 37% and 38% of patients without moderate to severe deterioration in FPS or lung function after SBRT

Study	nbr	Dose/fraction	Immbolisation of image guidance	Median follow-up	toxicity
Lagerwaard et al. [16]	219	100 Gy/5 60 Gy/5 60 Gy/8	4DCT	12	Late >or = grade 3 pneumonitis: 3% rib fracture: 1.8% (4; all in high dose area near chest wall) Chronic thoracic pain syndrome in 3 pts
Le et al. [17]	32 (11 meta)	30-40 Gy / 3-4	CyberKnife	21	Grade 3–5: 12.5% (3/4 with central lesions), all with dose >20 Gy 3 Grade 5, all central lesion: tracheal-esophageal fistula, pneumonitis, pleural effusion, pulmonary embolism and recalled pneumonitis
McGarry et al. [18]	47	42 Gy/3	Stereotactic Body Frame vacuum pillow		3/5 Patients who received 24 Gy/3 fractions developed Pgrade 3 toxicity in tumors >5 cm
Onimaru et al. [19]	45	48-60 Gy/6-7,5 Gy		17	1 Grade 1 esophagitis, later died of esophageal ulcer related bleeding from the same area of esophagitis
Song et al. [20]	32	40-60 Gy	Body frame	26.5	No >grade 2 pulmonary toxicity in peripheral tumors; 3/9 Centrally located tumors with Pgrade 3 pulmonary toxicity 1 Death from bleeding, aspiration and pneumonia due to complete bronchial stricture after 48 Gy/4 fractions
Xia et al. [21]	43	50 Gy/5	body gamma knife	54	Grade 2–3 pneumonitis: 4.6% (COPD prior to SBRT)
Zimmermann et al. [22]	68	24-40 Gy/3-5	vacuum couch and low pressure foil	17	6.4% Grade 3 pneumonitis after >12 months; 5% Rib fracture; 3.4% soft tissue fibrosis; 3.4% benign pleural effusion

Table 1. (Continued)

Study	nbr	Dose/fraction	Immbolisation of image guidance	Median follow-up	toxicity
Van der Voot. [23]	70	35–60 Gy/3	gold markers, CyberKnife	15	Late grade 3 toxicity was observed in seven patients (10%). Three patients had radiation pneumonitis. Four patients had thoracic pain requiring morfine
Guckenberger et al. [24]	124	37.5 Gy/3 26 Gy/1 48/6 Gy	stereotactic body frame, BodyFix system abdominal compression, 4DCT	18	Only 1 grade 3 pneumonitis Grade 3: 0.6% (esophageal ulceration)
Onimaru et al. [25]	28	48 Gy/4 40 Gy/4	gold markers		2 Grade 3 pneumonitis, both with poor pulmonary function prior to SBRT
Timmerman [26]	55	54 Gy/3	4D CT fluoroscopy. Respiration gating	34,4	Grade 3=24% grade 4= 4%
Hassbeek [27]	193	60 Gy/3/5/8	Novalis Brailab Exatrac	12.6	Late grade 3 pneumonitis 2.1%, rib fracture 3(1.6%), chronic chest pain 5 (2.6%)
Ricardi [28]	62	45 Gy/3	Elekta Precise SBF	28	Grade 3 radiation pneumonitis 2pts Rib fracture 1 pt, Chronic thorax pain 3 (4.8%).

Study	nbr	Dose/fraction	Immbolisation of image guidance	Median follow-up	toxicity
Gomez [29]	114	Médian dose 24 Gy	Clinac 2100EX, OBI, Cradle	10,7	Grades 3 and 4 (oesophageal toxicity 1 each). Grade 3 (bronchial toxicity) 1
Videtic [30]	26	50 Gy/5	IMRT-based SBRT Novalis ExacTrac vacuum bag	30,9	Acute grade 3 dyspnoea 1 (3.4%), Late chest pain Grade 2: 1(3.4%)
Brown [31]	31	60-67.5 Gy/3-5	CyberKnife, RTS	27,5	No grade 3 radiation pneumonitis 4, Oesophagitis 1
Stephans [32]	84	50 Gy/5	NA	NA	Grade 2 pneumonitis 2 (2.2%). Grade 2 chest late toxicity 9 (10%)
Soliman [33]	118	48-52 Gy/ 12-13	NA	23,8	Pneumonitis requiring steroids 5, late rib fracture 4

Although their functional impact is typically minimal, the lung parenchymal changes that are frequently observed on follow-up chest CTs present additional concern [49]. Trovo et al. described a radiographic lung injury pattern after SBRT. Their most common findings were diffuse or patchy ground-glass opacities that usually developed 2-6 months after treatment and a modified conventional pattern that included consolidation, volume loss, and bronchiectasis in the late period. Patients who did not have any radiological findings 6 weeks after treatment were more commonly found to have late grade 2-4 emphysema. No correlation could have been done with these radiologic patterns and known dose-volume histogram or normal tissue complication probability parameters [50].

The RP rates in Table 2 ranged from 9.4-28.0%. These variations may be due to each study's use of different planning target volumes (PTV), dose fractionation schedules, and RP scoring systems. Tucker et al. explored different scoring systems in a retrospective study of 442 patients who received definitive radiotherapy for NSCLC using three RP grading systems. Grade 2 or higher RP was observed in 129 (29%), 109 (25%), and 195 (44%) patients, according to the scoring systems of the Radiation Therapy Oncology Group (RTOG), Common Toxicity Criteria (CTC) v.2, and Common Terminology Criteria for Adverse Events (CTCAE) v.3 [52]. These results are consistent with the higher rate of RP that was observed in a study that used CTCA3 and 4 [37, 40, 42, 44]

Indiana University recently published one of the largest pooled analyses to investigate correlations between mean lung dose (MLD) (< 4 Gy vs. > 4 Gy), lung V20 (< 4% vs. > 4%) and grade 2–4 RP among patients treated with SBRT to total doses of 42–60 Gy given in 8-20 Gy fractions [41]. No grade 4-5 RP was observed by Chang et al. Grade 3 RP was experienced by only 3 patients (2.3%). Inappropriate cases of grade 3 RP were excluded and, when normal tissue dose volume constraints were respected, no difference in RP between central and peripheral lesions was proved. Interestingly, multivariate analysis found that RP was only associated with the amount of MLD in the ipsilateral lung. Specifically, the 14 patients (21.5% of the 65 patients) who had an ipsilateral lung MLD of ≥ 9.14 Gy had grade 2-3 RP. In contrast, only 1 patient (1.5% of the 65 patients) who had an ipsilateral lung MLD of < 9.14 Gy had grade 2-3 RP ($p < 0.001$) [43]. Consistent with the Chang et al. study [43], Guckenberger et al. also reported a link between the MLD of the irradiated ipsilateral lung and SBRT-induced RP [24]. Matsuo et al. found that a V25 of 4.2% or higher after SBRT was associated with a 50% risk of symptomatic RP [44]. The same study also reported that a PTV of > 37.7 cc was an independent predictive factor for grade 2 or higher RP [44]. If different dose regimens are used, the specific dose cutoffs may also differ. In RTOG 0236 and 0618 trials, the lung constraint parameter that was chosen to predict grade 2 or higher RP was a V20 of < 10%.

Based on experiences from Borst et al. [34] and Barriger et al. [41], it seems reasonable to limit MLD to 4–8 Gy in order to accept a < 10% risk of grade 2 or higher RP. Some biologic factors have been investigated to predict the risk of pneumonitis after SBRT. Hara et al. evaluated 16 patients who received a single-fraction SBRT dose of 20-35 Gy [53]. The occurrence of grade 3 RP (according to the RTOG criteria) was significantly correlated with the relative increase in the serum Krebs von den Lungen-6 (KL-6) between, before, and 2 months after SBRT.

A univariate analysis by Iwata et al. found that symptomatic RP was correlated with pretreatment serum KL-6 levels, gender, and PTV volume. Their multivariate analysis discovered that only the pretreatment KL-6 levels were significant [54]. Careful follow-up is necessary for patients with a pretreatment KL-6 level of ≥ 300 U/ml. CT or x-ray imaging before and after SBRT should help predict severe RP. In order to limit the risks of severe RP, Yamashita et al. recommended using a CT to prescreen for interstitial pneumonitis and also checking the serum KL-6 and surfactant protein-D (SP-D) levels. They reported that after prescreening was introduced, the rate of grade 4-5 RP decreased from 18.8% to 3.5% [55].

Unfit Patients

Patients who have comorbidities that currently prevent them from receiving surgery can be treated with SBRT. Most of these patients have cardiac morbidity or chronic obstructive pulmonary disease (COPD). COPD is classified according to The Global Initiative for Chronic Obstructive Lung Disease (GOLD); patients with COPD of grade III or IV (according to GOLD criteria) are considered to have severe COPD. These high-risk patients with severe COPD are known to have an 11-19% greater risk of death due to non-cancer causes.

Table 2. Summary of reports on dose–volume factors associated with radiation pneumonitis grade 2 or worse after stereotactic body radiation therapy

	Numb. of patients	Dose fractionation	Folllow-up (month)	RP grade 2 or worse	Suggested factors
Yamashita [37]	25	48 Gy/4–6 fr	-	28.0%	CI
Ricardi [39]	60	45 Gy/3 fr or 26 Gy/1 fr	-	14.3%	MLD 2 Gy eq (ipsilateral lung-CTV)
Borst [34]	128	35–60 Gy/4–8 fr	16,1	10.9%	MLD† (bilateral lung-GTV)
Guckenberger [24]	59	26 Gy/1 fr or 37.5 Gy/3 fr	13	18.6%	MLD and V2.5–50 (ipsilateral lung-CTV)
Ong [40]	18	55 Gy/5 fr or 60 Gy/8 fr	-	27.8%	total lung V5 >37 % and contralateral lung V5 >26 %
Barriger [41]	251	24–66 Gy/3–5 fr	-	9.4%	MLD >4 Gy and V20 >4% (bilateral lung-GTV)
Stauder [42]	84	32–60 Gy/3–5 fr	-	12.5%	PTV maximal dose
Matsuo [44]	74	48 Gy/4 fr	31,4	20.3%	PTV volume and V25 (bilateral lung-PTV)
Chang [43]	130	50 Gy /4 fr	26	12,6%	MLD ≥9.14 Gy (ipsilateral lung – GTV)
Baker [45]	263	-	15,6	11%	female gender, pack-years smoking, and larger GITV and PTV
Takeda [51]	265		19.2	23,6%	Heavy smoking was the strongest negative predictor for severe RP and was correlated with severe COPD.
Liu [38]	62 previously undergone conventional thoracic radiation therapy.	50 Gy /4 fr	16	20.8%	ECOG PS scores of 2-3 before SBRT FEV1≤65% before SBRT, V20≥30% of the composite (RT+SBRT) plan (P=.021), initial PTV in the bilateral mediastinum

A few studies have investigated SBRT's role in treating this patient with severe COPD [47, 48, 56]. In the Stephans et al. study, 92 consecutive patients who were undergoing SBRT for stage I lung cancer were evaluated by tests of forced expiratory volume at 1 second (FEV1) and a diffusion capacity to carbon monoxide (DLCO) before and at 6 months or more after SBRT. There was no significant overall change in the ability to predict the pulmonary function test results after SBRT; individual patients experienced both substantial improvements and declines. Nor did any factors improve the prediction of individual changes in the DLCO test.

However, the conformality index, V5, and V10 were associated with individual patient changes in FEV1% ($p = 0.033$, $p = 0.0036$, and $p = 0.025$, respectively) [48]. A study by Henderson et al. found that decreased baseline pulmonary function testing results (FEV1 and DLCO) were not associated with decreased 2-year survival. They also concluded that DLCO is "the most useful" pulmonary function testing to follow up lung injury caused by radiation [47]. However, Ohashi et al. reported that a small group of Japanese patients that received SBRT did not show any change in FEV1 but did have an increase in DLCO [56]. A study by Palma et al.'s evaluated the outcomes of SBRT on 176 patients with COPD GOLD III-IV and stage I NSCLC and performed a systematic review of the literature on outcomes after SBRT or surgery in these patients. They found that the mean 30-day mortality was 10% after surgery and 0% after SBRT. After both treatments, the rate of local or loco-regional control was high: 89%. However, after SBRT the overall survival rate was 79-95% at 1 year but declined to 43-70% at 3 years [57]. Mathematical modelling replicated similar findings [58]. It is not known if adverse events happened at a lower or higher rate in groups with COPD GOLD III-IV.

In contrast, for patients with severe COPD or a predicted postoperative (ppo) ppo-FEV1 of 40%, the evidence suggests that surgery would lead to high postoperative complications, high mortality rates, and risks to the patient's ability to resume independent living [59]. Additionally, severe COPD with poor pulmonary function should not be considered as a contraindication for SBRT [48, 57].

III. Chest Wall Toxicity

Chest wall (CW) toxicity may include a variety of adverse events such as rib fractures (table 3), CW pain (table 4), and skin changes. In some cases, patients may have pleural effusions associated with their CW pain. The reported incidence of CW toxicity ranges from 10-44% [40, 60-68]. Severe CW pain that requires narcotic analgesia has been reported in approximately 1-2% of patients [26, 32, 64, 66]. In contrast, after lobectomy, thoracotomic pain syndromes occur in about 50% of patients [69]. After 4 to 5 years, 30% of patients still experience this pain [70]. Although the majority of postsurgical patients have mild to moderate pain, up to 10% of them experience severe and disabling pain [71]. However, video-assisted thoracoscopic surgery seems to lead to better outcomes and less severe pain in the postoperative setting [72]. Creach et al. and Andolino et al. found that the median time to rib fracture was longer than the median time to isolated CW pain, 19.2 vs. 8.9 months [73] and 13.5 vs. 6 months [60], respectively. Their pathophysiology are likely to be different.

Risk factors for developing CW pain include the treatment volume and distance of the tumor from the CW. In a retrospective study, 265 patients (268 tumors) had tumors ≤ 2.5 cm from the CW. This study found that 104 of these patients (39%) developed skin toxicity (any grade), 14 (5%) reported acute pain (any grade), and 45 (17%) had chronic pain. Body mass index (BMI) was also strongly associated with the development of CW pain patients with a BMI of > 29 had almost twice the risk of chronic pain ($p = 0.03$). Among patients with a BMI of > 29, diabetes mellitus was a significant contributing factor in the development of chest pain [62]. Stephans et al. found a trend toward CW pain in patients who continued to be active smokers at the time of treatment [61].

The V30 has frequently been reported as a significant risk factor for the development of CW pain. However, studies that used varied dose and fractionation schedules found that cut off values varied from 30-70 cm^3 [61, 62, 64, 67, 73]. Dunlap et al. [64] demonstrated that the volume of CW that receives > 30 Gy predicts the risk of developing severe pain and/or rib fracture after lung SBRT. They thus recommend that the volume of CW that will receive 30 Gy should be limited, if possible, to no more than 10 cm^3. In order to limit the risk of CW pain to < 15% of patients, Creach et al. proposed that the V30 and V40 be < 0.7% and 0.19%, respectively [73]. Stephans et al. reported that the V30 to ≤ 30 cm^3 of the CW and the V60 to ≤ 3 cm^3 of the CW should result in a 10-15% (or lower) risk of late CW toxicity [61]. Andolino et al. emphasized that high dose can predict CW toxicity and thus stated that the maximum dose delivery should be 50 Gy in 3-5 fractions to the V40 (<5 cm^3) and V60 (≤ 3 cm^3) [60].

However, as increasingly large tumors are being treated with SBRT, the reported incidence of CW toxicity may also increase [40]. Various lung studies that evaluated a relatively small number of patients found that the rates of rib fractures ranged from 3-42.4% [60, 62, 64, 74-78]. Some of these studies included asymptomatic rib fractures [60, 64, 77, 78]. The proximity of the tumor to the CW influenced the development of rib fractures. Several studies also found that the incidence of rib fracture increased in conjunction with the proportion of peripheral lesions. In a study in which 88% of lung lesions were peripheral, Nambu et al. reported a 2-year actuarial incidence of rib fracture of 27.4% [76].

In a study where only peripheral tumors were included, Voroney et al. [75] discovered a 2-year actuarial incidence of rib fracture 21.4%. And for tumors located near (< 1 cm) the chest-wall, Kim et al. saw a 2-year actuarial incidence of rib fracture of 42.4% [78]. The use of a CT to detect rib fractures increased the rate of their incidence [76, 78].

In contrast, studies that included lesions from all locations in the CW, within 2.5 cm of the CW [64], or in which the 50% isodose line abutted the CW [60], reported a rib fracture rate of 2.7–8.3%. Few studies have investigated rib fractures and their dosimetric correlation [74, 77]. However, Pettersson et al. did specifically examine how radiation dose affects the development of rib fractures after SBRT [74]. They found the strongest association of rib fracture in the small-volume/high-dose regions of the CW. In a study of 116 patients, Asai et al. found that 24.1% of them had a rib fracture (according to a CT) and 10.34% had been symptomatic. Factors that are significantly associated with a risk of rib fractures include a maximum dose (Dmax) of 42.4 Gy, V40 of > 0.29 cc, V30 of > 1.35 cc, and V20 of > 3.62 cc [77].

Kim et al. suggested that most of the patients developed rib fractures were elderly and the lifetime risk of osteoporosis-related fractures in women was 3.3 times higher than that in men. This difference can explain why rib fracture following SBRT occurred more frequently in females than in males (2-year fracture rate of 64.7% vs. 33.7%, respectively; $p = 0.0140$) [78].

Table 3. Reported rib fracture

Author	Nb pt	Peripherical tumor %	Follow up	(CT/symptomatic)	Suggested factors
Pettersson [74]	68	-	29	16%	the 5% and 50% risks are given by D2cm3 = 3 × 9.1 Gy and 3 × 16.6 Gy, respectively.
Voroney [75]	42	100% ?		21.4%	
Nambu [76]	177	88%	27	23.2% (CT)/ 7,9% symptomatic	-
Kim [78]	296	40%	22	42.4% (CT)	-
Andolino [60]	311	59%	19	5,7%	D max 50 Gy
Asai [77]	116	-	-	24.1% (CT)/ 10,34% symptomatic	Rib fractures—Dmax 42.4 Gy V40 >0.29 cc V30 >1.35 cc V20 >3.62 cc

Table 4. Studies on chest wall toxicities with dosimetric correlation

Study	Nb patient	Dose fractionation	Follow up (month)	Suggested factors
Pettersson et al. [74]	68	45 Gy/3	29	Rib fractures—D2cc of \ 21 Gy, 27.3 Gy, and 49.8 Gy: 0 %, 5 %, and 50 %
Dunlap et al. [64]	60	21–60 Gy/3-5	11,1	A 30% risk of developing severe CW toxicity correlated with a V30 >35 cc
Andolino et al. [60]	311	54 Gy (18–72 Gy)/2-5	19	Chest wall pain and/or rib fractures Dmax : Cutoff at 50 Gy 5 cc and 15 cc of CW receiving 40 Gy predict a 10% and 30% risk of CW toxicity, respectively.
Welsh et al. [62]	265	50 Gy/4	10,3	V30 >30 cc versus <30 cc: 18 % versus 2.7 %
Mutter et al. [67]	126	40–60 Gy/ 3–5	16	V30 >70 cc
Stephans et al. [61]	45	60 Gy/3	18.8	Skin changes, chest wall pain, and/or rib fracture V30 >30 cc and V60 >3 cc
Creach et al. [73]	140	54 Gy/3 50 Gy/5	22,5	V30 threshold of 0.7% and V40 threshold of 0.19% was correlated with a 15% risk of CW pain.

IV. Esophageal Toxicity

A study by Onimaru et al. (48 Gy/8 fractions) reported that a 4 cm length of esophagus was included in the 80% isodose area with a maximum dose of 50.5 Gy. The radiation-induced esophagitis that resulted led to bleeding and 1 death [25]. A Stanford University study investigated spine or lung tumors that were < 1 cm from the esophagus and received single- or multiple-fraction SBRT. The 3 esophageal toxicity events that occurred included esophagitis (grade 2), tracheoesophageal fistula (grade 4–5), and esophageal perforation (grade 4–5). The dosimetric parameters that were examined included the D5cc, D2cc, D1cc, and Dmax with the linear-quadratic model. The D5cc, D2cc, D1cc, and Dmax for the 3 patients ranged from 10.7–16.5 Gy, 13.7–18.2 Gy, 15.7–19 Gy, and 18.5–22.8 Gy, respectively [79].

V. Bronchial Toxicity

Although a few cases of bronchial complications have been reported after chest SBRT, dosimetric analysis is lacking. In terms of toxicities, however, a patient that was enrolled in a Phase I trial of SBRT for stage I medically inoperable NSCLC and treated to 72 Gy in 3 fractions was observed with tracheal necrosis [18]. Joyner et al. also found that a prescribed and delivered dose of 36 Gy in 3 fractions was followed by bronchial occlusion [80]. And a series from South Korea reported that 8 of the 9 patients that had centrally located lung tumours that were treated to 40–60 Gy in 3–4 fractions developed partial or complete bronchial structure [20]. A study from the Memorial Sloan-Kettering Cancer Center (MSKCC), which treated 114 patients (119 para-spinal sites) with single-dose SBRT of 18–24 Gy, observed 2 cases of grade 2 or 3 bronchial toxicity. The D1cc were 11.01 Gy (cough) and 22.11 Gy (bronchial stenosis), respectively [29]. Corradetti et al. recently reported that a patient received an SBRT regimen of 50 Gy in 5 fractions to a centrally located lung tumor and, 8 months later, developed a case of fatal central-airway necrosis with hemoptysis [81]. The maximum airway dose was limited to no more than 52.5 Gy in 5 fractions.

VI. Other Toxicities

Other toxicities, such as soft-tissue fibrosis [82], skin reaction [83], and brachial plexopathy, [84] have also been observed. However, these toxicities occur in < 1% of treated patients and changes in treatment planning can prevent their occurrence.

Brachial Plexopathy

Brachial plexus injury should also be considered if the tumor is at the apex of a lung. Per directions in RTOG 0236, the ipsilateral axillary/subclavian vessels were used as a surrogate for the brachial plexus for the major trunks of the brachial plexus. After a median of 7 months (range, 6-23 months), grades 2-4 brachial plexopathy developed in 7 out of 36 patients. The 2-year risk of brachial plexopathy for the maximum brachial plexus dose of > 26 Gy was 46% vs. 8% for a dose of ≤ 26 Gy. The authors concluded that the maximum dose to the brachial plexus should be kept at < 26 Gy in 3-4 fractions [84].

Skin Toxicity

Hoppe et al. [83], examined the risk factors associated with severe skin toxicities in 50 patients with stage I NSCLC who were treated to 60 Gy in 3 fractions or 44-48 Gy in 4 fractions. Risk factors for grade 2 or higher acute skin toxicity were found to be the use of only 3 beams, a < 5 cm distance between the tumor and the skin of the posterior CW, and a maximum skin dose of ≥ 50% of the prescribed dose. However, the maximum skin dose was not associated with skin toxicities in locations other than the back and the bolus effect of immobilization devices has been suspected [83]. A Welsh et al. study reported that the volume of the CW that received 30 Gy in 4 fractions predicted the risk of skin toxicity among patients with lung tumours ≤ 2.5 cm cm of the CW [62]. RTOG protocols require that the skin, which is defined as a 5 mm concentric ring beneath the body contour surface, receive single-fraction SBRT at 23 Gy (< 10 cc) and 26 Gy (< 0.03 cc).

Conclusion

Dose tolerances were generally determined from retrospective chart reviews (that were directly derived from outcomes) or via mathematical modelling. Dose tolerance isn't determined by prospectively compiling dose and volume information from Phase I trials in which the only manipulated variable was the dose. Phase II trial information can be analyzed, but comparing outcomes between centers is potentially problematic due to differences in patient selection, treatment conduct (including dosimetry principles), and follow-up scrutiny. Furthermore, additional multicenter trials are needed to corroborate the results from single-institution trials. Longer-term follow-up is also required to assess late toxicities from SBRT.

Given the concerns regarding severe late effects, the tolerance information that is related to SBRT would ideally be gathered from a more formal and rigorous process than the trial-and-error approach that has historically been used for conventionally fractionated radiotherapy.

One complicating factor that many study authors identified is that the apparently similar nominal radiation dose prescriptions that are reported across a series can actually represent widely varying dose intensities. Future publications on SBRT should thus use standardized dose reporting and specify how targets were defined, what dose was delivered to both the target's periphery and center, how the dose conformed, and which dose calculation algorithm was used. Algorithms that do not accurately model radiation interactions in tissues of heterogeneous density (particularly in the lung) should be phased out due to their unpredictable and potentially great misrepresentation of the actual delivered doses [85]. Similarly, it will be important to standardize how local progression is assessed and distinguished from treatment-related pulmonary changes.

References

[1] Palma, D; Senan, S. Stereotactic radiation therapy: changing treatment paradigms for stage I nonsmall cell lung cancer. *Curr Opin Oncol*, 2011, 23, 133-9.

[2] Baumann, P; Nyman, J; Lax, I; et al. Factors important for efficacy of stereotactic body radiotherapy of medically inoperable stage I lung

cancer. A retrospective analysis of patients treated in the Nordic countries. *Acta Oncol*, 2006, 45, 787–95.

[3] Baumann, P; Nyman, J; Hoyer, M; et al. Outcome in a prospective phase II trial of medically inoperable stage I non-small-cell lung cancer patients treated with stereotactic body radiotherapy. *J Clin Oncol*, 2009, 27, 3290–6.

[4] Fakiris, A; McGarry, R; Yiannoutsos, C; et al. Stereotactic body radiation therapy for early-stage non-small-cell lung carcinoma: four-year results of a prospective phase II study. *Int J Radiat Oncol Biol Phys*, 2009, 75, 677–82.

[5] Kopek, N; Paludan, M; Peterson, J; et al. Stereotactic body radiotherapy for medically inoperable stage I non-small cell lung cancer: mature outcome, toxicity results. *Int J Radiat Oncol Biol Phys*, 2008, 72, S37.

[6] Koto, M; Takai, Y; Ogawa, Y; et al. A phase II study on stereotactic body radiotherapy for stage I non-small cell lung cancer. *Radiother Oncol*, 2007, 85, 429–34.

[7] Nagata, Y; Takayama, K; Matsuo, Y; et al. Clinical outcome of a phase I/II study of 48 Gy of stereotactic body radiotherapy in 4 fractions for primary lung cancer using a stereotactic body frame. *Int J Radiat Oncol Biol Phys*, 2005, 63, 1427–31.

[8] Onishi, H; Shirato, H; Nagata, Y; et al. Hypofractionated stereotactic radiotherapy (HypoFXSRT) for stage I non-small cell lung cancer: updated results of 257 patients in a Japanese multi-institutional study. *J Thorac Oncol*, 2007, 2, S94–S100.

[9] Salazar, O; Sandhu, T; Lattin, P; et al. Once-weekly, high-dose stereotactic body radiotherapy for lung cancer: 6-year analysis of 60 early-stage, 42 locally advanced, and 7 metastatic lung cancers. *Int J Radiat Oncol Biol Phys*, 2008, 72, 707–15.

[10] Takeda, A; Sanuki, N; Kunieda, E; et al. Stereotactic body radiotherapy for primary lung cancer at a dose of 50 Gy total in five fractions to the periphery of the planning target volume calculated using a superposition algorithm. *Int J Radiat Oncol Biol Phys*, 2009, 73, 442–8.

[11] Uematsu, M; Tukui, T; Tahara, K; et al. Long-term results of computed tomography guided hypofractionated stereotactic radiotherapy for stage I non-small cell lung cancers. *Int J Radiat Oncol Biol Phys*, 2008, 72, S37.

[12] Chang, J; Balter, P; Dong, L; et al. Stereotactic body radiation therapy in centrally and superiorly located stage I or isolated recurrent non-small-cell lung cancer. *Int J Radiat Oncol Biol Phys*, 2008, 72, 967–71.

[13] Collins, B; Vahdat, S; Erickson, K; et al. Radical Cyberknife radiosurgery with tumor tracking: an effective treatment for inoperable small peripheral stage I non-small cell lung cancer. *J Hematol Oncol*, 2009, 2, 1.

[14] Fritz, P; Kraus, H; Blaschke, T; et al. Stereotactic, high single-dose irradiation of stage I non-small cell lung cancer (NSCLC) using four-dimensional CT scans for treatment planning. *Lung Cancer*, 2008, 60, 193–9.

[15] Hoyer, M; Roed, H; Hansen, A; et al. Prospective study on stereotactic radiotherapy of limited-stage non-small-cell lung cancer. *Int J Radiat Oncol Biol Phys*, 2006, 66, S128–35.

[16] Lagerwaard, F; Haasbeek, C; Smit, E; et al. Outcomes of risk-adapted fractionated stereotactic radiotherapy for stage I non-small-cell lung cancer. *Int J Radiat Oncol Biol Phys*, 2008, 70, 685–92.

[17] Le, Q; Loo, B; Ho, A; et al. Results of a phase I dose–escalation study using single-fraction stereotactic radiotherapy for lung tumors. *J Thorac Oncol*, 2006, 1, 802–9.

[18] McGarry, R; Papiez, L; Williams, M; et al. Stereotactic body radiation therapy of early-stage non-small-cell lung carcinoma: phase I study *Int J Radiat Oncol Biol Phys*, 2005, 63, 1010–5.

[19] Onimaru, R; Shirato, H; Shimizu, S; et al. Tolerance of organs at risk in small-volume, hypofractionated, image-guided radiotherapy for primary and metastatic lung cancers. *Int J Radiat Oncol Biol Phys*, 2003, 56, 126–35.

[20] Song, S; Choi, W; Shin, S; et al. Fractionated stereotactic body radiation therapy for medically inoperable stage I lung cancer adjacent to central large bronchus. *Lung Cancer*, 2009, 66, 89–93.

[21] Xia, T; Li, H; Sun, Q; et al. Promising clinical outcome of stereotactic body radiation therapy for patients with inoperable stage I/II non-small-cell lung cancer. *Int J Radiat Oncol Biol Phys*, 2006, 66, 117–25.

[22] Zimmermann, F; Geinitz, H; Schill, S; et al. Stereotactic hypofractionated radiotherapy in stage I (T1-2N0M0) non-small-cell lung cancer (NSCLC). *Acta Oncol*, 2006, 45, 796–801.

[23] Van der Voort Van Zyp, N; Prévost, J; Hoogeman, M; et al. Stereotactic radiotherapy with real-time tumor tracking for non-small cell lung cancer: clinical outcome. *Radiother Oncol*, 2009, 91, 296–300.

[24] Guckenberger, M; Wulf, J; Mueller, G; et al. Dose–response relationship for image-guided stereotactic body radiotherapy of pulmonary tumors:

relevance of 4D dose calculation. *Int J Radiat Oncol Biol Phys*, 2009, 74, 47–54.

[25] Onimaru, R; Fujino, M; Yamazaki, K; et al. Steep dose–response relationship for stage I non-small-cell lung cancer using hypofractionated high-dose irradiation by real-timetumor-trackingradiotherapy. *Int J Radiat Oncol Biol Phys*, 2008, 70, 374–81.

[26] Timmerman, R; Paulus, R; Galvin, J; et al. Stereotactic body radiation therapy for inoperable early stage lung cancer. *JAMA*, 2010, 303, 1070–6.

[27] Haasbeek, C; Lagerwaard, F; Antonisse, M; et al. Stage I nonsmall cell lung cancer in patients aged > or = 75 years : outcomes after stereotactic radiotherapy. *Cancer*, 2010, 116, 406-14.

[28] Ricardi, U; Filippi, A; Guarneri, A; et al. Stereotactic body radiation therapy for early stage non-small cell lung cancer: results of a prospective trial. *Lung Cancer*, 2010, 68, 72-7.

[29] Gomez, D; Hunt, M; Jackson, A; et al. Low rate of thoracic toxicity in palliative paraspinal single-fraction stereotactic body radiation therapy. *Radiother Oncol*, 2009, 93, 414-8.

[30] Videtic, G; Stephans, K; Reddy, C; et al. Intensity-modulated radiotherapy-based stereotactic body radiotherapy for medically inoperable early-stage lung cancer: excellent local control. *Int J Radiat Oncol Biol Phys*, 2010, 344-9.

[31] Brown, W; Wu, X; Fayad, F; et al. Application of robotic stereotactic radiotherapy to peripheral stage I non-small cell lung cancer with curative intent. *Clin Oncol*, 2009, 21, 623-31.

[32] Stephans, K; Djemil, T; Reddy, C; et al. A comparison of two stereotactic body radiation fractionation schedules for medically inoperable stage I non-small cell lung cancer: the Cleveland Clinic experience. *J Thorac Oncol*, 2009, 4, 976–82.

[33] Soliman, H; Cheung, P; Yeung, L; et al. Accelerated hypofractionated radiotherapy for early-stage non-small-cell lung cancer: long-term results. *Int J Radiat Oncol Biol Phys*, 2011, 79(2), 459-65.

[34] Borst, G; Ishikawa, M; Nijkamp, J; et al. Radiation pneumonitis in patients treated for malignant pulmonary lesions with hypofractionated radiation therapy. *Radiother Oncol*, 2009, 91, 307-13.

[35] Bishawi, M; Kim, B; Moore, W; et al. Pulmonary function testing after stereotactic body radiotherapy to the lung. *Int J Radiat Oncol Biol Phys*, 2012, 82, 107-10.

[36] Takeda, A; Ohashi, T; Kunieda, E; et al. Early graphical appearance of radiation pneumonitis correlates with the severity of radiation pneumonitis after stereotactic body radiotherapy (SBRT) in patients with lung tumors. *Int J Radiat Oncol Biol Phys*, 2010, 77, 685-90.

[37] Yamashita, H; Nakagawa, K; Nakamura, N; et al. Exceptionally high incidence of symptomatic grade 2-5 radiation pneumonitis after stereotactic radiation therapy for lung tumors. *Radiat Oncol*, 2007, 2, 21.

[38] Liu, H; Zhang, X; Vinogradskiy, Y; et al. Predicting radiation pneumonitis after stereotactic ablative radiation therapy in patients previously treated with conventional thoracic radiation therapy. *Int J Radiat Oncol Biol Phys*, 2012, 84(4), 1017-23.

[39] Ricardi, U; Filippi, A; Guarneri, A; et al. Dosimetric predictors of radiation-induced lung injury in stereotactic body radiation therapy. *Acta Oncol*, 2009, 48, 571-7.

[40] Ong, C; Palma, D; Verbakel, W; et al. Treatment of large stage I-II lung tumors using stereotactic body radiotherapy: Planning considerations and early toxicity. *Radiother Oncol*, 2010, 97, 431-6.

[41] Barriger, R; Forquer, J; Brabham, J; et al. A dose-volume analysis of radiation pneumonitis in non-small cell lung cancer patients treated with stereotactic body radiation therapy *Int J Radiat Oncol Biol Phys*, 2012, 82, 457-62.

[42] Stauder, M; Macdonald, O; Olivier, K; et al. Early pulmonary toxicity following lung stereotactic body radiation therapy delivered in consecutive daily fractions. *Radiother Oncol*, 2011, 99, 166-71.

[43] Chang, J; Liu, H; Balter, P; et al. Clinical outcome and predictors of survival and pneumonitis after stereotactic ablative radiotherapy for stage I non-small cell lung cancer. *Radiation Oncology*, 2012, 7, 152

[44] Matsuo, Y; Shibuya, K; Nakamura, M; et al. Dose–Volume Metrics Associated With Radiation Pneumonitis After Stereotactic Body Radiation Therapy for Lung Cancer. *Int J Radiation Oncol Biol Phys*, 2012, 83(4), 545-9.

[45] Baker, R; Han, G; Sarangkasiri, S; et al. Clinical and Dosimetric Predictors of Radiation Pneumonitis in a Large Series of Patients Treated With Stereotactic Body Radiation Therapy to the Lung *Int J Radiation Oncol Biol Phys*, 2013, 85(1), 190-5.

[46] Guckenberger, M; Kestin, L; Hope, A et al. Is there a lower limit of pretreatment pulmonary function for safe and effective stereotactic body radiotherapy for early-stage non-small cell lung cancer? *J Thorac Oncol*, 2012, 7, 542–51.

[47] Henderson, M; McGarry, R; Yiannoutsos, C; et al. Baseline pulmonary function as a predictor for survival and decline in pulmonary function over time in patients undergoing stereotactic body radiotherapy for the treatment of stage I non-small-cell lung cancer. *Int J Radiat Oncol Biol Phys*, 2008, 72, 404–9.

[48] Stephans, K; Djemil, T; Reddy, C; et al. Comprehensive analysis of pulmonary function test (PFT) changes after stereotactic body radiotherapy (SBRT) for stage I lung cancer in medically inoperable patients *J Thorac Oncol*, 2009, 4, 838-44.

[49] Bradley, J. Radiographic response and clinical toxicity following SBRT for stage I lung cancer. *J Thorac Oncol*, 2007, 2, S118–S24.

[50] Trovo, M; Linda, A; Naqa, I; et al. Early and late lung radiographic injury following stereotactic body radiation therapy (SBRT). *Lung Cancer*, 2010, 69(1), 77-85.

[51] Takeda, A; Kunieda, E; Ohashi, T; et al. Severe COPD is correlated with mild radiation pneumonitis following stereotactic body radiotherapy. *Chest*, 2012, 141(4), 858-66.

[52] Tucker, S; Jin, H; Wei, X; et al. Impact of toxicity grade and scoring system on the relationship between mean lung dose and risk of radiation pneumonitis in a large cohort of patients with non-small cell lung cancer. *Int J Radiat Oncol Biol Phys*, 2010, 77, 691-8.

[53] Hara, R; Itami, J; Komiyama, T; et al. Serum levels of KL- 6 for predicting the occurrence of radiation pneumonitis after stereotactic radiotherapy for lung tumors. *Chest*, 2004, 125, 340-4.

[54] Iwata, H; Shibamoto, Y; Baba, F; et al. Correlation between the serum KL-6 level and the grade of radiation pneumonitis after stereotactic body radiotherapy for stage I lung cancer or small lung metastasis. *Radiother Oncol*, 2011, 101, 267-70.

[55] Yamashita, H; Kobayashi-Shibata, S; Terahara, A; et al. Prescreening based on the presence of CT-scan abnormalities and biomarkers (KL-6 and SP-D) may reduce severe radiation pneumonitis after stereotactic radiotherapy. *Radiat Oncol*, 2010, 5, 32.

[56] Ohashi, T; Takeda, A; Shigematsu, N; et al. Differences in pulmonary function before vs. 1 year after hypofractionated stereotactic radiotherapy for small peripheral lung tumors. *Int J Radiat Oncol Biol Phys*, 2005, 62, 1003–8.

[57] Palma, D; Lagerwaard, F; Rodrigues, G. Curative treatment of stage I non-small-cell lung cancer in patients with severe COPD: stereotactic

radiotherapy outcomes and systematic review. *Int J Radiat Oncol Biol Phys*, 2012, 82, 1149–56.

[58] Louie, A; Rodrigues, G; Hannouf, M; et al. Withholding stereotactic radiotherapy in elderly patients with stage I non-small cell lung cancer and co-existing COPD is not justified: outcomes of a Markov model analysis *Radiother Oncol*, 2011, 99(2), 161-5.

[59] Finlayson, E; Fan, Z; Birkmeyer, J. Outcomes in octogenarians undergoing high-risk cancer operation: a national study. *J Am Coll Surg*, 2007, 205, 729-34.

[60] Andolino, D; Forquer, J; Henderson, M; et al. Chestwall toxicity after stereotactic body radiotherapy for malignant lesions of the lung and liver. *Int J Radiat Oncol Biol Phys*, 2011, 80, 692–7.

[61] Stephans, K; Djemil, T; Tendulkar, R; et al. Prediction of Chest Wall Toxicity From Lung Stereotactic Body Radiotherapy (SBRT). *Int J Radiat Oncol Biol Phys*, 2012, 82, 974–80.

[62] Welsh, J; Thomas, J; Shah, D; et al. Obesity increases the risk of chest wall pain from thoracic stereotactic body radiation therapy *Int J Radiat Oncol Biol Phys*, 2011, 81(1), 91–6.

[63] Bongers, E; Haasbeek, C; Lagerwaard, F; et al. Incidence and risk factors for chest wall toxicity after risk-adapted stereotactic radiotherapy for early-stage lung cancer. *J Thorac Oncol*, 2011, 6, 2052-7.

[64] Dunlap, N; Cai, J; Biedermann, G; et al. Chest wall volume receiving >30 Gy predicts risk of severe pain and/or rib fracture after lung stereotactic body radiotherapy *Int J Radiat Oncol Biol Phys*, 2010, 76, 796–801.

[65] Chi, A; Liao, Z; Nguyen, N; et al. Systemic review of the patterns of failure following stereotactic body radiation therapy in early-stage non-small-cell lung cancer: clinical implications. *Radiother Oncol*, 2010, 94, 1-11.

[66] Andratschke, N; Zimmermann, F; Boehm, E; et al. Stereotactic radiotherapy of histologically proven inoperable stage I non-small cell lung cancer: patterns of failure. *Radiother Onco*, 2011, 101, 245–9.

[67] Mutter, R; Abreu, A; Jackson, A; et al. Predictors of chest wall toxicity following stereotactic body radiotherapy for early stage non-small cell lung cancer. *Oncology*, 2010, 24, 12 [Abstract].

[68] Stephans, K; Woody, N; Videtic, G; et al. Chest wall toxicity from lung sterotactic body radiotherapy (SBRT): a dosimetric analysis using several fraction schemes. *Int J Radiat Oncol Biol Phys*, 2010, 75, 506 [Abstract].

[69] Rogers, M; Duffy, J. Surgical aspects of chronic post-thoracotomy pain. *Eur J Cardiothorac Surg*, 2000, 18, 711-6.

[70] Karmakar, M; Ho, A. Postthoracotomy pain syndrome. *Thorac Surg Clin*. 2004, 14, 345-52.

[71] Kehlet, H; Jensen, T; Woolf, C. Persistent postsurgical pain: *risk factors and prevention Lancet* 2006, 367, 1618 –25.

[72] Wildgaard, K; Ravn, J; Nikolajsen, L; et al. Consequences of persistent pain after lung cancer surgery: a nationwide questionnaire study. *Acta Anaesthesiol Scand*, 2011, 55, 60 – 8.

[73] Creach, KM; et al. Dosimetric predictors of chest wall pain after lung stereotactic body radiotherapy. *Radiotherapy and Oncology*, 2012, 104, 23–7

[74] Pettersson, N; Nyman, J; Johansson, K. Radiation-induced rib fractures after hypofractionated stereotactic body radiation therapy of non-small cell lung cancer: adose-andvolumeresponseanalysis. *Radiother Oncol*, 2009, 91, 360–8.

[75] Voroney, J; Hope, A; Dahele, M; et al. Chest wall pain and rib fracture after stereotactic radiotherapy for peripheral non-small cell lung cancer. *J Thorac Oncol*, 2009, 4, 1035–7.

[76] Nambu, A; Onishi, H; Aoki, S; et al. Rib fracture after stereotactic radiotherapy on follow-up thin-section computed tomography in 177 primary lung cancer patients. *Radiat Oncol*, 2011, 6, 137.

[77] Asai, K; Shioyama, Y; Nakamura, K; et al. Radiation-induced rib fractures after hypofractionated stereotactic body radiation therapy: risk factors and dose-volume relationship. *Int J Radiat Oncol Biol Phys*, 2012 84(3), 768–73.

[78] Kim, S; Song, S; Kwak, J; et al. Clinical prognostic factors and grading system for rib fracture following stereotactic body radiation therapy (SBRT) in patients with peripheral lung tumors. *Lung Cancer*, 2013, 79(2), 161–6.

[79] Abelson, J; Murphy, J; Loo, B; et al. Esophageal tolerance to high-dose stereotactic ablative radiotherapy. *Diseases of the Esophagus*, 2012, 25(7), 623–9.

[80] Joyner, M; Salter, BJ; Papanikolaou, N; et al. Stereotactic body radiation therapy for centrally located lung lesions *Acta Oncol*, 2006, 45, 802–7.

[81] Corradetti, M; Haas, A; Rengan, R. Central-airway necrosis after stereotactic body-radiation therapy. *N Engl J Med*, 2012, 366(24), 2327–9.

[82] Kawase, T; Takeda, A; Kunieda, E; et al. Extrapulmonary soft-tissue fibrosis resulting from hypofractionated stereotactic body radiotherapy for pulmonary nodular lesions. *Int J Radiat Oncol Biol Phys*, 2009, 74(2), 349-54.

[83] Hoppe, B; Laser, B; Kowalski, A; et al. Acute skin toxicity following stereotactic body radiation therapy for stage I non-small-cell lung cancer: who's at risk? *Int J Radiat Oncol Biol Phys*, 2008 72(5), 1283-6.

[84] Forquer, J; Fakiris, A; Timmerman, R; et al. Brachial plexopathy from stereotactic body radiotherapy in early-stage NSCLC: dose-limiting toxicity in apical tumor sites *Radiother Oncol*, 2009, 93(3), 408-13.

[85] Xiao, Y; Papiez, L; Paulus, R; et al. Dosimetric evaluation of heterogeneity corrections for RTOG 0236: stereotactic body radiotherapy of inoperable stage I-II non-small-cell lung cancer *Int J Radiat Oncol Biol Phys*, 2009, 73, 1235-42.

In: The Revolution of Robotic …
Editor: Pierre-Yves Bondiau
ISBN: 978-1-62808-718-5

Chapter 16

Other Local Treatments

Pierre-Yves Bondiau*
Department of Radiation Oncology,
Antoine-Lacassagne Cancer Center, Nice, France
University of Nice Sophia-Antipolis, Nice, France

Abstract

The treatment of choice for NSCLC at an early stage is a lobectomy. 20-25% of patients with early-stage NSCLC are poor candidates for lobectomy because of concomitant severe cardiac or pulmonary comorbidities or the patient refuses surgery. For these patients, conventional radiotherapy with 60 to 70 Gy delivered in 30-35 fractions over a period of 6-7 weeks usually leads to poor survival rates at 3 years (20-40%) and 5 years (10-30%).

In this chapter, we will present a short review of the literature regarding alternative treatment options for this cohort of patients.

Pattern of Recurrence after SBRT

A retrospective analysis of recurrence after SBRT was presented by Senthi [1] of 676 patients with a median follow-up of 32·9 months. 124 (18%)

* Email: pierre-yves.bondiau@nice.unicancer.fr.

patients had disease recurrence. Actuarial 2-year rates of local, regional, and distant recurrence were 4·9%, 7·8%, and 14·7%, respectively. Corresponding 5-year rates of local, regional, and distant recurrence were 10·5%, 12·7%, and 19·9%, respectively. 82 (66%) were distant recurrences and 57 (46%) were isolated distant recurrences. Isolated locoregional recurrences occurred in the remaining 42 patients with disease recurrence (34%), 35 (83%) of whom did not develop subsequent distant recurrence. In this study, new pulmonary lesions characterised as second primary tumours in the lung developed in 6%at a median of 18·0 months after SBRT. The conclusions were that late recurrences after SBRT are infrequent with two unique patterns. The predominant pattern is out-of-field, isolated distant recurrence presenting early, despite initial PET staging. A second, less prevalent pattern is that patients develop isolated locoregional recurrences 33% of the time.

Radiofrequency and Microwaves or SBRT

These treatments induce heat in the tissue by raising ionic stirring for RF and microwave motion of water molecules to the microwaves. They are electromagnetic currents from 300 to 500 kHz frequency to the radio frequency from 900 to 2450 MHz for the microwave. The treatment with RF probe (Cf. Figure 1) needs plates dispersion of the patient (circuit) while this is not necessary with the microwave. For radio frequency, it needs from 20 to 30 minutes to coagulate a tumor of 3 cm diameter. The microwave option causes a faster heating time, which can reduce treatment time by half. In a review of 219 studies, Bilal [2] shows that RFQ and SBRT have improved survival rates compared with conventional RT. Results for overall survival and local control are presented in Table 1. In this review, complications for RFQ included: pneumothorax (19.1-63%). Primary complications for SBRT included: Fatigue (31-32.6%), pneumonitis (2.1-12.5%) and pain (3.1-12%). The author finds a higher recurrence rate after RFQ.

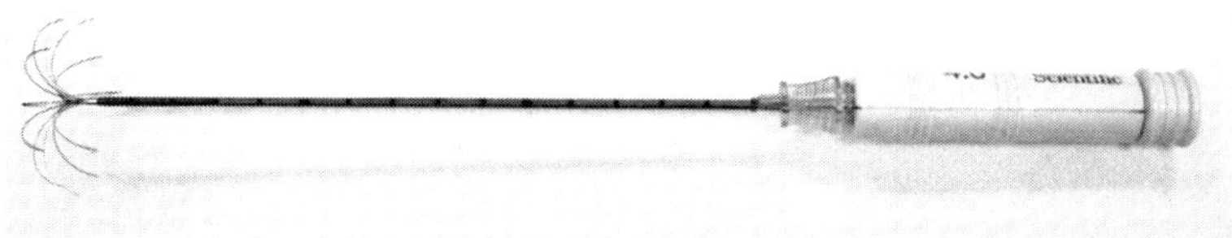

Figure 1. Radiofrequency probe.

Table 1. Results for overall survival and local control

		RFQ	SBRT
Overall survival	1 year	68.2–95%	81–85.7%
	3 years	36–87.5%	42.7–56%
	5 years	20.1–27%	47%
Local control		3.5–14.5%	23.7–43%

Renaud [3] performed a retrospective analyses of 202 studies in which23 show a clear advantage for SBRT. The current published studies show that SBRT is a safe and effective procedure and should be proposed first to patients suffering from primary NSCLC unfit for surgery. But as there is no blind, prospective control, randomized study comparing these techniques, these preliminary results must be interpreted with caution.

Photodynamic Therapy

Photodynamic therapy (PDT) produces a delayed necrosis of tumor cells by the combined action of a photosensitizing agent (which makes the cells sensitive to light), light and oxygen present in the cells. It may be used to treat very early stage lung cancers that are still confined to the outer layers of the lung airways when other treatments aren't appropriate or to clear an airway obstruction in the case of advanced cancer. PDT can also be used to help open up airways blocked by tumors to improving breathing. For this technique, a light-activated drug called porfimer sodium is injected into a vein. This drug is more likely to collect in cancer cells than in normal cells. After a couple of days (to give the drug time to build up in the cancer cells), a bronchoscope is passed down the throat and into the lung. A special laser light on the end of the bronchoscope is directed to the tumor, which activates the drug and causes cell necrosis. A possible side effect to this therapy is sensitivity to light.

Laser Therapy

Lasers can be used to treat very small lung cancers in the linings of airways. Laser resection is conducted with a bronchoscope (rigid endoscope) under general anesthesia. It can be used in the case of lung cancer to help quickly clear the trachea or a large bronchus to improve breathing. This technique can also be used to help open up airways blocked by larger tumors to help people breathe better.

Cryotherapy

Cryosurgery is the application of extreme cold to destroy abnormal or diseased tissue. The cryoprobe is located in the tumor, and then the freezing occurs under pressure of argon through the circulation in the probe. The Joule-Thomson effect discloses that the temperature decreases as the gas expands. From -20 ° C, cell death occurs by destruction of cell membranes and protein denaturation. To achieve the most complete destruction possible, it is important to create a thermal shock with several phases: a freezing phase with argon, then thawing and freezing again with argon. This freeze-thaw-freeze cycle creates cytotoxic temperatures (less than -20°C to -40°C) that encompass the entire anticipated tumor volume. The entire process takes approximately 30 minutes. Patients undergo CT-guided percutaneous thoracic cryotherapy over 2 hours under local or general anesthesia. This technique is under clinical evaluation.

Stent Placement

Lung tumors that have grown into an airway can sometimes cause trouble breathing or other problems. To help keep the airway open (often after other treatments such as PDT or laser therapy), a hard silicone or metal tube called a stent may be placed in the airway using a bronchoscope.

Conclusion: SBRT vs. Surgery?

In the near future, some surgical techniques could be discussed in terms of efficiency and cost. In a study presented by Lagerwaard [4] the outcomes after SBRT were analyzed in patients with potentially operable stage I NSCLC. The median follow-up was 31.5 months; and median overall survival was 61.5 months. OS rates at 3 years in patients with (n = 59) and without (n = 118) histological diagnosis were 96% versus 81%. Post-SABR 30-day mortality was 0%. Local control rates at 1 and 3 years were 98% and 93%, respectively. Toxicity was mild, with grade ≥3 radiation pneumonitis and rib fractures in 2% and 3%, respectively.

This study supports ongoing randomized clinical trials comparing surgery and SBRT in cases of operable stage I NSCLC.

References

[1] Senthi S, Lagerwaard FJ, Haasbeek CJ, Slotman BJ, Senan S. Patterns of disease recurrence after stereotactic ablative radiotherapy for early stage non-small-cell lung cancer: a retrospective analysis. *Lancet Oncol.* 2012 Aug;13(8):802-9.

[2] Bilal H, Mahmood S, Rajashanker B, Shah R. Is radiofrequency ablation more effective than stereotactic ablative radiotherapy in patients with early stage medically inoperable non-small cell lung cancer? *Interact Cardiovasc Thorac Surg.* 2012 Aug;15(2):258-65.

[3] Renaud S, Falcoz PE, Olland A, Massard G. Is radiofrequency ablation or stereotactic ablative radiotherapy the best treatment for radically treatable primary lung cancer unfit for surgery? *Interact Cardiovasc Thorac Surg*. 2013 Jan;16(1):68-73.

[4] Lagerwaard FJ, Verstegen NE, Haasbeek CJ, Slotman BJ, Paul MA, Smit EF, Senan S. Outcomes of stereotactic ablative radiotherapy in patients with potentially operable stage I non-small cell lung cancer. *J Radiat Oncol Biol Phys*. 2012 May 1;83(1):348-53. doi: 10.1016/j.ijrobp.2011.06.2003. Epub 2011 Nov 19.

Part IV: Conclusion

In: The Revolution of Robotic …
Editor: Pierre-Yves Bondiau
ISBN: 978-1-62808-718-5

Conclusion

Pierre-Yves Bondiau[1,2]
[1]Department of Radiation Oncology, Antoine-Lacassagne Cancer Center, Nice, France
[2]University of Nice Sophia-Antipolis, Nice, France

Progress since the first pneumonectomy has been constant in all areas; diagnosis, staging, treatment modalities, and therapeutic strategies. But results are not at an expected level. The hope for improving treatment outcomes lies in screening for early diagnosis, but also by decreasing the risk of recurrence. Irradiation techniques currently being developed allow to deliver high dose of radiation, named SBRT. SBRT allows to decrease the risk of recurrence and conduces to new way to think the treatment of lung cancer. Moreover, rSBRT with CK can track the tumor during irradiation, leading to a drastic decrease of PTV. In function of the location of the tumor in the lung, direct detection of tumor's contrast is possible. In others cases, fiducial's insertion is mandatory. Different types of fiducials can be used, and if tumor is not moving with the breathing, direct bone-based contrast detection can be used.

Presents indication of SBRT for Primitive tumors can be summarized: Stage I medically inoperable or Patients stage I who refuse surgery, Stage III for a boost (research or after clinical case discussion), Lung tumor reirradiation, Recurrence on unique lung. For lung secondary tumors the indication is oligo metastatic patients with a slow growing tumor profile. It can be used for pain metastasis, obstructing endobronchial lesion and clinical research. The delivery of precisely targeted radiation doses to lung tumors in a hypofractionated fashion is feasible and safe. Image-guided robotic stereotactic radiosurgery of pulmonary metastases with the CK achieves good rates of local disease control with limited toxicity to surrounding tissues and in many cases may be beneficial for patients for whom surgery is not an option. Impressive late locoregional control rates and the existence of long-term and disease-free survivors is demonstrated.

Another recent study has estimated cancer risk per unit mass of irradiated normal tissue based on integral dose calculation and the observed secondary cancer incidence in a cohort of 5000 survivors of childhood cancer [41]. It has been shown that the risk increases with the dose and the irradiated mass (volume). Compared to conventional radiotherapy, the volume receiving a dose higher than 40 Gy (high risk per unit dose) is smaller with SBRT, and the volume receiving a dose lower than 5 Gy (low risk per unit dose) is larger. Therefore, the risks are balanced on each side. In addition, it is worth noting that the volume receiving an ablative dose cannot develop secondary cancer, due to total cell kill. Taken together, it is unlikely that SBRT will lead to more secondary cancers than conventional radiotherapy.

The results indicate that the delivery of precisely targeted ablative radiation doses with surgical precision to limited treatment volumes of lung tumors in a hypofractionated fashion is feasible and safe. Image-guided robotic stereotactic radiosurgery of lung tumors with CyberKnife achieves excellent rates of local disease control with limited toxicity to surrounding tissues and, in many cases, might be curative for patients for whom surgery is not an option.

The revolution is underway and prompts us to use CK to treat high-risk but operable patients whose only surgical treatment option is wedge resection.

Part V: Annexes

In: The Revolution of Robotic …
Editor: Pierre-Yves Bondiau
ISBN: 978-1-62808-718-5

Annex A: List of Abbreviations

3DRT	Tri-dimension radiotherapy
2DRT	Two-dimension radiotherapy
AJCC	American Joint Committee on Cancer
BED	Biologic Equivalent Dose
BMI	Body Mass Index
BPC	Bronchopulmonary cancer
BPCB	Bronchoscopic protected catheter brush
CK	CyberKnife
COPD	chronic obstructive pulmonary disease
CSS	Cause-Specific Survival
CT	Computed Tomography
CTC	Common Toxicity Criteria
CTV	Clinical Target Volume
CVC	Central venous catheter
CW	Chest Wall
DRR	Digitally Reconstructed Radiograph
EBUS	Endobronchial Ultrasound
ENB	Electromagnetic navigation bronchoscopy
FEV	Forced Expiratory Volume
FM	Fiducial Marker
FSU	Functional SubUnits
GOLD	Global initiative for Chronic Obstructive Lung Disease
GTV	Gross Target Volume
HU	Hounsfield unit
IASLC	International Association for the Study of Lung Cancer
KL-6	Krebs von den Lungen-6

LED	Luminescent Electronic Device
LQ	linear quadratic
LR	Local Recurrence
LRR	LocoRegional recurrence
MLC	Multi Leaf Collimator
MLD	Mean Lung Dose
MU	Monitor Units
NSCLC	Non Small Cell Lung Cancer
NTCP	Normal Tissue Complication Probability
OAR	Organ At Risk
OS	Overall Survival
PDT	Photodynamic therapy
PDU	Power Down Unit
PET	Positron Emission Tomography
PET/CT	Positron Emission Tomography and CT scan
PS	Performance status
PTV	Planified Treatment Volume
RFA	Radiofrequency ablation
RFA	Radiofrequency Ablation
RP	Radiation Pneumonitis
RR	Regional Recurrence
rSBRT	robotic Stereotactic Body RadioTherapy
RTOG	Radiation Therapy Oncology Group
SBRT	Stereotactic Body RadioTherapy
SCLC	Small Cell Lung Cancer
SEER	Surveillance, Epidemiology, and End Results Program
TCP	Tumor Control Probability
TNM	Tumor, Node, Metastases
VT	Videothoracoscopy
XLTS	XSight Lung Tracking System
XSP	Xsight Spine

In: The Revolution of Robotic …
Editor: Pierre-Yves Bondiau
ISBN: 978-1-62808-718-5

Annex B: Margins for Cyberknife Treatment

Table of margins with Method A or Method B

Method A

	Software	GTV-CTV mm	CTV-PTV mm
Lung primitive	Fiducial X-lung X-spine	5 5 5	2 2 2AP, 2LR, 5HF
Metastasis	Fiducial X-lung X-spine	0 0 0	2 2 2AP, 2LR, 5HF

Method B

	Software	GTV-PTV mm
Lung tumors	any	5

In some case margins can be adapted in case of proximity of OAR.

In: The Revolution of Robotic …
Editor: Pierre-Yves Bondiau

ISBN: 978-1-62808-718-5

Annex C: Organ at Risk Constraint

Fraction		1		3		5	
	(1) Vol max (cc)	max (Gy)/ Vol(1)	Max (Gy)	max (Gy)/ Vol(1)	Max (Gy)	max (Gy)/ Vol(1)	Max (Gy)
Spinal cord	0,25	8	14	18	21	22,5	30
Brachial Plexus	3	14,4	14	22,5	24	30	32
	3	14,4		22,5	24	30	32
Œsophagus	5	11		17	25	19	35
Vessels	10	31	16	39	45	47	53
Heart	15	16	16	24	30	32	38
Trachea/ bronchus	4	8,8	10	15	30	18	
Skin	10	14,4	23	22,5	33	30	
	Critical Volume	dose max/VC		dose max/VC		dose max/VC	
Lung (R)	1500	7		10		12,5	
Lung (L)	1000	7,4		11,4		13,5	

In: The Revolution of Robotic …
Editor: Pierre-Yves Bondiau
ISBN: 978-1-62808-718-5

Annex D: Patient Positioning

1. Before Dosimetric Modality

A vacuum mattress is made before dosimetric CT scan or dosimetric PET/CT:

- Patient is set into a vacuum mattress
- In comfortable and natural position
- Arms along the body
- A mark (m) on the mattress is made near the position of the tumor
- Dosimetric modality is made (annex E,F)

2. Prepositioning

As the synchrony software is used, the patient is prepared with the "synchrony shirt".

- He is installed into the vacuum mattress.
- A manual set-up (centimetric) is made with the help of laser onto the mark (m)

3. Positioning

A. Tumor Track during Breathing Active

1. Fiducial Inserted

- A first set-up is made by XRay with the spine to detect migration in case of fiducial
- Then, a second set-up is made on the fiducial
- synchrony software is started

2. Direct Contrast Tracking with Xsight Lung Software

- A first set-up is made by the software onto the spine then, a second set-up is made with the contrast of the tumor
- synchrony software is started

B. No Tumor Tracking

- Patient is installed into the vacuum mattress.
- A manual set-up is made with the help of laser
- infra millimetric Set-up is made with xsight spine software

In: The Revolution of Robotic …
Editor: Pierre-Yves Bondiau
ISBN: 978-1-62808-718-5

Annex E: Dosimetric CT Scan Characteristics

- The positioning of the patient in a vacuum mattress is made with a specific CK pallet
- CT is performed in free breathing.

CT acquisition parameters in our Center are the following:

- Slice thickness: 1.25 mm
- Slice increment: continuous
- Helicoidal acquisition
- Resolution matrix: 512x512
- Pitch: 1.75
- Rotation time: 0.8 s
- Field of View ≥ 500 mm
- Number of slices < 512
- Tube current and exposure time: 100-150 mAs (Use of dose reduction software)
- Tube voltage: 120 kV (Use of dose reduction software)

Delineation

1) Delineation of GTV is made on level 500 HU / window 500 HU
2) Delineation of OAR is made in relation with the position of the tumor in the lung
3) Delineation of OAR (cf. annexe C) at less than 3 cm from GTV in our Center

In: The Revolution of Robotic …
Editor: Pierre-Yves Bondiau
ISBN: 978-1-62808-718-5

Annex F: Dosimetric PET/CT System Characteristics

- PET systems are most commonly hybrid PET/CT. These systems combine a whole-body PET and a multi-slice CT.
- For dosimetric use, a laser system is installed in front of the PET/CT gantry to define the isocentre. In order to use its full capacities, full-dose PET/CT is recommended for RT planning. Some centers may even use iodine-contrast media. In our center and in CK planning, we use full-dose PET/CT from the top of the vertex down to the pubic symphysis, but no contrast.

Image acquisition

- Images are acquired in the same manner as in a RT simulation procedure using the same immobilization material as used for positioning the patient such as a body vacuum bag and positioning lasers.
- Patients are positioned on a specific CK pallet that is mounted on a flat carbon fiber RT pallet, mounted itself on top of the PET/CT patient pallet.
- Since CK treatment is delivered during normal breathing, non-gated PET/CT data are sufficient even if SUV can be underestimated. Different gating systems are however available when needed.
- PET/CT are performed in free breathing.
- CT acquisition parameters in our Center are the following:
    - Slice thickness: 1mm

  - Slice increment: continuous
  - Resolution matrix: 512x512
  - Pitch: 1
  - Rotation time: 1s
  - Field of View $\geq$ 550 mm
  - Number of slices < 500
  - Tube current and exposure time: 100-150 mAs (Use of dose reduction software)
  - Tube voltage: 100-120 kV (Use of dose reduction software)
- FDG-PET acquisition parameters in our Center are the following:
  - FDG activity injected: 3 MBq/kg
  - Beds: Number of beds according to CT (7-8), 150s per bed
  - Matrix: 256x256
  - Acquisition mode 3D, static
  - Iterative reconstruction: 2 iterations, 21 subsets
  - Images are corrected for random coincidences, scatter and attenuation using CT data
  - Smoothing with a Gaussian filter (FWHM = 5mm)

Target volume selection

- Staging lung cancer with FDG-PET is more accurate than with CT (NSCLC & SCLC) avoiding unnecessary treatment.
- PET/CT influences the GTV. Volumes are reduced when FDG-negative lymph nodes are excluded.

Target volume delineation

- FDG-PET has a positive impact on radiation therapy planning notably by having a better inter-observer reproducibility.
- FDG-PET is more accurate in delineating heterogeneous tumor or within an atelectasis area.
- FDG-PET detects areas of tumor where boosts can be delineated.

The main limit is the absence of standardization in tumoral segmenting methods.

Editor's Contact Information

Pierre-Yves Bondiau, M.D., Ph.D.
Head of Cyberknife/Cyclotron Unit
Centre Antoine Lacassagne
227 av de la Laterne
06200 Nice, France
Tel: +33 4 92 03 12 61
pierre-yves.bondiau@nice.unicancer.fr

Index

#

A

B

C

N

O

P

T

U

V

W

X